# Breaths of life :

# The daily life of a

# *Caregiver*

# *in*

# *Pneumology*

*MARTIN STERLING*

*« In pulmonology, every breath counts. It's a department where we learn to listen to the breath of life, to watch out for its fragility, and to accompany each patient towards freer breathing. »*

# Table of contents

# Chapter 11: Respiratory rehabilitation and the role of the caregiver

## Chapter 12: Pain management in pneumology     323

## Chapter 13: The role of the caregiver in the care of patients with rare respiratory diseases

## Chapter 14: Care of patients with respiratory disabilities      393

# Chapter 1

# Introduction to Pneumology

- **The pulmonology specialty: Definition and role of the department**
  - Respiratory conditions treated (asthma, COPD, pneumonia, bronchial cancer, etc.)

Respiratory diseases treated in pulmonology cover a wide range of pathologies affecting the respiratory system, each with its own particularities in terms of diagnosis, management and patient support. Some of these conditions, such as asthma, chronic obstructive pulmonary disease (COPD), pneumonia and bronchial cancer, are common and well-known, while others are rarer and require a more specialized approach.

**Asthma**, for example, is a chronic disease characterized by inflammation of the airways, leading to bronchial hyperreactivity. Asthma attacks are marked by episodes of respiratory discomfort, wheezing and coughing, often exacerbated by allergens, infections or physical exertion. Asthma management is based on background treatment with inhaled corticosteroids and, in the event of an attack, the administration of bronchodilators to rapidly relieve symptoms. Caregivers play a key role in monitoring asthma patients, in particular by ensuring the correct use of inhalation devices and identifying the warning signs of an attack.

COPD, another major respiratory pathology, is often the result of prolonged exposure to tobacco or pollutants. It is characterized by progressive and irreversible airway obstruction, associated with chronic inflammation. COPD patients generally suffer from dyspnea, chronic cough and copious bronchial secretions. Their management includes bronchodilators, inhaled corticosteroids and, in some cases, long-term oxygen therapy. In this context, the caregiver must carefully monitor the patient's respiratory function, assess signs of decompensation and provide support with daily activities, as respiratory fatigue can limit patients' autonomy.

**Pneumonia** is a lung infection of bacterial, viral or fungal origin. They manifest as a productive cough, fever, chest pain and respiratory distress. Pneumonia can vary in severity, from mild forms to cases requiring hospitalization or even respiratory assistance. Treatment is based on the administration of antibiotics or antivirals, depending on the cause, as well as supportive measures such as oxygen therapy. The caregiver's role is crucial in monitoring vital parameters, watching for signs of sepsis or respiratory distress, and preventing complications, notably by mobilizing the patient early to avoid complications associated with bed rest.

**Bronchial cancer**, or lung cancer, is one of the most feared pathologies in pulmonology. There are different types of bronchial cancer, the most common being non-small-cell and small-cell carcinomas. Symptoms, often delayed, include persistent cough, haemoptysis, weight loss and progressive dyspnoea. Treatment of bronchial cancer depends on the stage, and may include surgery, radiotherapy, chemotherapy or immunotherapy. Supporting patients with bronchial cancer goes beyond simply administering treatment. The caregiver must offer constant support, both physically and emotionally, accompanying the patient through palliative care if necessary, while ensuring comfort and quality of life.

In addition to these common conditions, the Pulmonology Department also treats rarer respiratory diseases such as pulmonary fibrosis, tuberculosis and pulmonary hypertension. Each of these diseases presents specific challenges in terms of management, and requires special attention from the care teams. For example, **pulmonary fibrosis** leads to thickening of lung tissue, making gas exchange difficult and causing severe dyspnea. Treatment of this condition relies on antifibrosis drugs, but monitoring and support by the caregiver are essential to manage the patient's fatigue and breathlessness.

In short, the respiratory diseases treated in pulmonology are varied, and each requires a tailored approach, both in terms of therapy and day-to-day patient care. The nursing auxiliary plays a central role in this care, providing clinical monitoring, comfort care and indispensable moral support to patients, who are often faced with chronic or serious illnesses that have a major impact on their quality of life.


        ◦   The importance of multidisciplinary management
Multidisciplinary management in respiratory medicine is essential to offer patients a comprehensive approach to care, adapted to the complexity of their pathologies. Respiratory diseases, whether acute or chronic, affect much more than the lungs: they affect the whole body, the quality of life, the psychological state, and often the social conditions of patients. This is why close collaboration between several health professionals is essential to ensure comprehensive, coordinated and effective care.

Pneumology, by its very nature, demands a wide range of skills and specific interventions that cannot be fully provided by a single discipline. As a specialist in respiratory diseases, the pulmonologist plays a central role in diagnosis and treatment. However, he or she relies on a wider team to implement day-to-day care. Care assistants, nurses, physiotherapists, dieticians, psychologists and social workers are all professionals who, together, form a support network for the patient.

**Nurses**, for example, are at the heart of the direct relationship with patients. They constantly monitor their clinical condition, assessing signs of respiratory distress and vital parameters, and helping to manage devices such as oxygen therapy. Their role is not limited to technical care, as they also provide psychological support by listening to the fears and needs of patients, who are often distressed by their respiratory difficulties. Working in close collaboration with nurses and doctors, orderlies ensure continuous monitoring of care, anticipating complications and responding rapidly to patients' changing needs.

**Nurses** play a key role in treatment management. They administer medication, adjust oxygen doses, and monitor examinations prescribed by doctors, such as blood gases or chest X-rays. Their collaboration with the nursing assistants is vital to the coordination of care, as each member of the team brings a different observation to bear on the evolution of the patient's condition. This synergy between nurses and orderlies is one of the pillars of multidisciplinary care.

Another key player is the **respiratory physiotherapist**, who intervenes to help patients improve their lung function, particularly in cases of chronic obstructive pulmonary disease (COPD) or after pneumonia. Respiratory physiotherapy helps to clear secretions, strengthen respiratory muscles and improve overall lung capacity. Rehabilitation exercises are particularly useful for patients in remission, or those suffering from chronic illnesses that affect their ability to breathe properly. The physiotherapist works in direct liaison with the nursing team to adapt his or her sessions to the patient's general condition, in order to avoid overexertion or complications. The nursing auxiliary takes part in these sessions, helping to mobilize the patient, ensuring comfort and closely monitoring the evolution of symptoms.

**Dieticians** are often called upon to adapt the diet of patients suffering from respiratory diseases. Dyspneic patients may find it difficult to eat properly, leading to weight loss and malnutrition. Poor nutrition has a direct impact on the body's ability to fight infection and maintain good muscular function, including the respiratory muscles. The dietician's role is therefore to suggest suitable diets, rich in proteins and calories, but easy for patients to consume. This nutritional management, although sometimes discreet, is crucial in helping patients recover and maintain their strength, particularly in the case of chronic pathologies.

Another often overlooked but fundamental aspect is psychological support. **Psychologists** play a vital role in managing anxiety and depression, two conditions frequently associated with chronic respiratory illness. Fear of suffocation, helplessness in the face of disease, or the impact of assisted ventilation on self-image are all factors that can weigh heavily on patients' morale. The intervention of a psychologist can give patients the tools they need to manage stress, accept their body's limitations and cope better with their illness. Communication between the medical team and the psychologist is essential to provide coherent, integrated care that takes into account the patient's emotional state, not just his or her physical state.

Finally, **social workers** are also key members of the multidisciplinary team. Their intervention is essential for patients needing help in organizing their discharge from hospital, support at home or referral to specialized services. They ensure that patients benefit from available social aid, home respiratory assistance devices, or an environment conducive to recovery or day-to-day disease management.

- **Role and responsibilities of the respiratory orderly**
  - The link between patient and care team

The relationship between patient and healthcare team is at the heart of quality care in pulmonology. This bond is fundamental, as it is based on a relationship of trust and continuous communication, which determines both the effectiveness of the care provided and the patient's well-being. In pneumology, where chronic or acute respiratory illnesses can have a major impact on the patient's daily life, this relationship becomes even more crucial, not least because of the respiratory vulnerability and anxiety associated with difficulty in breathing. The care team, made up of nursing assistants, nurses, doctors and other professionals, must create an environment in which the patient feels listened to, supported and involved in his or her care.

From the moment they are admitted to the respiratory department, patients are often confronted with a medicalized environment that can be a source of anxiety, due to the presence of respiratory equipment such as oxygen masks, ventilators or monitoring devices. In this situation, the first contact with the care team plays a decisive role. Caregivers, with their constant proximity to the

24

patient, are often the first to establish this relationship. They take charge of everyday tasks, making sure that the patient is comfortable, and ensuring that his or her basic needs are met. These seemingly simple interactions - helping to wash, feed and mobilize - are in fact key moments when a human bond is forged, and the patient begins to trust the team around him or her.

The nursing auxiliary, through its regular presence at the patient's bedside, often becomes the privileged interlocutor for expressing concerns, discomforts or simply practical needs. They are also the ones who most closely observe the evolution of the patient's clinical condition, detecting early signs of deterioration, such as increased respiratory rate, cyanosis, or a drop in oxygen saturation. This vigilance, combined with attentive listening to the patient's complaints, enables rapid reaction, often in consultation with nurses and doctors. In this way, the nursing auxiliary acts as a bridge between the patient and the rest of the care team, transmitting essential information that enables treatments or care to be adjusted according to the patient's actual condition.

In this relationship, communication is essential. It's not limited to the technical aspects of care, but also encompasses the emotional dimension. Breathing is a vital act, and any difficulty in breathing naturally generates feelings of fear, even panic. The role of the nursing team is to provide not only medical answers, but also psychological support. With reassuring words, clear explanations and a calming presence, caregivers help to reduce the patient's anxiety. Their ability to simply explain complex ,procedures such as the installation of an oxygen therapy device or the need for a fibroscopy, helps patients to better understand their situation and cooperate in their care.

The relationship between patient and care team is not limited to verbal exchanges. It also includes respect for the patient's autonomy. Involving patients in decisions concerning their care is a key factor in establishing a relationship of trust. When patients understand and consent to proposed treatments, and are encouraged to ask questions or express their preferences, they become active players in their own health. For example, a patient suffering from COPD can, in consultation with the team, decide the best time for a respiratory physiotherapy session, depending on how tired he or she is. In this context, the caregiver can play a facilitating role, relaying the patient's needs and requests to other team members.

The multidisciplinary nature of the respiratory care team also strengthens this bond with the patient. Each professional brings his or her own specific expertise to the table, but it is through the unity and coordination of their actions that the patient experiences comprehensive, coherent care. Exchanges between orderlies, nurses, physiotherapists and doctors must be fluid, so that the patient perceives that his or her condition is being monitored from different angles. This increases their sense of security and confidence, as they know that their well-being is being taken care of at all levels.

This bond between patient and care team is also important at the most difficult times, such as during respiratory decompensation or at the end of life. Respiratory distress, particularly in serious pathologies such as pulmonary fibrosis or advanced bronchial cancer, is a deeply distressing experience. In these situations, the support of the nursing team becomes essential to accompany the patient, not only on a medical level, but also in a human and compassionate dimension. The caregiver, by virtue of his or her proximity and role as first point of contact, is often the one who guides the patient through these critical moments, providing a comforting presence, physical support to ease discomfort, and a constant link with other healthcare professionals to adjust care.

○    Working in pairs with the nurse and doctor
Caregivers, nurses and doctors working in pairs are an essential part of respiratory patient care, enabling efficient coordination of care and guaranteeing a tailored response to the complex needs of respiratory patients. This partnership is based on a clear, yet

flexible, division of roles, where each contributes his or her specific skills, while working closely together to ensure continuity of care. This two-way working relationship, between the caregiver and the nurse on the one hand, and between these two and the doctor on the other, is based on communication, trust and constant sharing of information.

The caregiver/nurse pair is at the heart of daily care. The caregiver is often the first to be in direct contact with the patient. He or she provides basic care, such as personal hygiene, feeding assistance, mobilization and monitoring vital signs. In this context, the caregiver doesn't just carry out assigned tasks: he or she carefully observes the patient's condition, detects subtle changes in breathing, appearance or behavior, and relays this crucial information to the nurse. This constant feedback between caregiver and nurse is fundamental to adjusting care in real time, anticipating possible complications and reacting rapidly when necessary.

Nurses, on the other hand, have a more technical and therapeutic vision of care, and their responsibilities include managing drug treatments, monitoring devices such as oxygen therapy or ventilators, and administering medical procedures under delegation from the doctor. In collaboration with the caregiver, the nurse takes into account the latter's observations to assess the effectiveness of ongoing treatments or to adjust certain interventions. For example, if the caregiver notices that the patient is showing signs of respiratory fatigue after a physiotherapy session, the nurse can adjust oxygen administration or reassess the frequency of respiratory treatments. In the same way, the caregiver can help prepare the patient for more technical care, facilitate the installation of equipment or even provide moral support to the patient during sometimes uncomfortable procedures.

Working in pairs is also crucial in emergency situations, where perfect coordination between caregiver and nurse enables rapid action to be taken. For example, in the case of acute respiratory distress, the caregiver may be the one who spots the first signs - sudden shortness of breath, cyanotic lips - and immediately calls the nurse to begin emergency interventions, such as administering oxygen or calling the doctor for further treatment. In these moments, trust between the two professionals, based on fluid communication and complementary skills, is crucial to saving lives.

The doctor, for his part, plays a more centralized role in diagnostic assessment, therapeutic decision-making and overall patient management. However, he or she cannot exercise this responsibility effectively without the support of the nursing assistant/nurse pair. Indeed, the doctor relies heavily on the information provided by the care team to refine his diagnoses and adapt treatments. During medical visits, the caregiver and nurse share their observations with the doctor: the quality of the patient's sleep, his tolerance of exertion, the evolution of his dyspnea, or details of the effectiveness of the treatments administered. These exchanges enable the doctor to make informed decisions, such as adjusting oxygen therapy, modifying a drug prescription or scheduling additional tests such as a chest scan or blood gas.

What's more, in the field of pulmonology, where many patients suffer from chronic diseases such as COPD or severe asthma, continuity of care is crucial. The doctor draws up a long-term treatment plan, but it's the caregiver/nurse duo who ensure its proper execution on a daily basis. They monitor response to treatment, support the patient in self-management activities such as the use of inhalers, and provide regular feedback to the doctor on the progress of the disease. In this context, the caregiver also plays the role of educator, supporting the patient to better understand his or her disease, explaining simple techniques to better manage breathing or the correct use of nebulization equipment.

The interaction between orderlies, nurses and doctors is not limited to clinical situations. It also takes place during team transmissions, key moments when each member shares the information gathered during his or her shift to ensure smooth care. During these transmissions, the orderly reports his or her detailed observations on the evolution of the patient's condition, while the nurse summarizes the technical interventions and treatments administered. The doctor, informed of these elements, can then adapt care protocols, suggest new tests or adjust current treatments. This team dynamic, reinforced by working closely in pairs, ensures that patients benefit from personalized care that is constantly adjusted to their needs.

   ◦   Helping patients with everyday tasks

Accompanying patients in their day-to-day activities is one of the most fundamental aspects of the caregiver's role, particularly in pneumology, where respiratory diseases directly affect patients' ability to perform simple, essential tasks. Conditions such as COPD, severe asthma, pneumonia or bronchial cancer often limit patients' ability to lead an active life, as breathing, a vital function, becomes a constant effort. This is where the caregiver comes in, helping the patient to regain a certain degree of autonomy and comfort in everyday gestures, while taking care to preserve their dignity and support their overall well-being.

In pneumology, dyspnea (difficulty in breathing) is a ubiquitous symptom that makes even the simplest tasks, such as getting up, washing or getting dressed, extremely exhausting. The caregiver accompanies the patient in these activities, providing physical support, but also psychological support to overcome the anxiety often linked to the sensation of breathlessness. For example, during toileting, a key moment in daily care, the caregiver must ensure that the patient is comfortably seated, often in a seated position, to avoid any deterioration in breathing. This means not only helping with personal hygiene, but also respecting the patient's rhythm, pausing if necessary to avoid exacerbating respiratory fatigue.

Helping patients with everyday tasks is based on careful observation of their state of health. Every day, the caregiver assesses the patient's physical capabilities and adapts his or her assistance according to changes in the patient's condition. A patient who, the day before, was able to get up on his own to go to the bathroom may need more help the next day if he is more tired or if his respiratory symptoms have worsened. This flexibility is essential to provide optimum support without compromising the patient's autonomy. The caregiver therefore plays a balancing role, intervening discreetly but effectively, encouraging the patient to participate actively in the actions he or she is capable of performing, while being ready to take over if necessary.

In addition to hygiene care, assistance with eating is another area where patient support becomes crucial. Many patients suffering from respiratory illnesses find it difficult to eat because of their shortness of breath. Chewing, swallowing and breathing become exhausting tasks, and some may fear false routes, particularly in the elderly or very weak. The caregiver must therefore be present to adapt the meal environment: seat the patient correctly, cut food if necessary, and above all ensure that the patient eats slowly and takes time to breathe between each mouthful. It is important to choose foods that are easy to chew and swallow, in collaboration with the dietician if necessary, to ensure adequate nutrition despite respiratory difficulties.

As part of mobilization, the caregiver also has a key role to play in preserving or improving the patient's physical capacity. Many pulmonary patients, especially those suffering from chronic diseases such as COPD, tend to limit their physical activity for fear of aggravating their dyspnea. However, prolonged immobility can lead to muscular degradation, cardiac complications and an increased risk of pulmonary infections. Support for mobilization must therefore be gradual and respectful of the patient's rhythm. The caregiver can encourage the patient to perform small exercises adapted to his or her abilities, such as sitting on the edge of the bed, getting up with assistance, or walking a few steps around the room. Every gesture, no matter how simple, contributes to maintaining a certain level of physical fitness and preventing the complications associated with prolonged bed rest, such as bedsores or infections.

In addition, the use of medical devices, such as oxygen therapy or assisted ventilation, is an integral part of the daily life of pneumology patients. Caregivers play a major role in helping patients to use and manage these devices, which can be a source of stress and discomfort. They ensure that the equipment is correctly installed, that the oxygen mask or goggles are correctly positioned, and teach the patient how to use the equipment independently whenever possible. This support not only ensures the effectiveness of the treatment, but also helps the patient to better accept these devices, which are often perceived as a constraint. The caregiver must also alert the patient to warning signals, such as choking or respiratory discomfort, which require rapid intervention by the nursing team.

Assisting patients with everyday tasks also has an important psychological dimension. Respiratory patients, particularly those with chronic illnesses, can feel dependent or frustrated by their inability to perform what were once simple tasks. The caregiver, by being present in a caring way, helps the patient to regain self-confidence, to accept his or her temporary or permanent limitations, and to focus on the progress made, however small. The caregiver's patience and active listening lighten the emotional burden of the disease, and provide vital moral support, especially when patients feel isolated or discouraged by their condition.

- **Introduction to breathing apparatus and devices**
  - Assisted ventilation, oxygen therapy, aerosols

**Assisted ventilation**, **oxygen therapy** and **aerosols** are essential therapeutic devices in pulmonology, designed to help patients breathe more easily or improve oxygen supply. These treatments are frequently used for patients with acute or chronic respiratory illnesses, such as COPD, severe asthma, pneumonia or respiratory failure. Each of these devices has a specific role to play in patient care, and requires particular attention from the nursing team, especially the orderlies who are in daily contact with these patients and these tools.

**Assisted ventilation** is a technique that helps or completely replaces the patient's breathing. It is used when the respiratory muscles are too weak to ensure efficient breathing, or when the patient's state of health no longer allows sufficient gas exchange between air and blood. There are two main types of assisted ventilation: invasive and non-invasive. Invasive ventilation involves intubation of the patient, often in an intensive care setting, where a tube is inserted into the trachea to connect the patient directly to a mechanical ventilator. This method is used in the most severe cases, where breathing has completely failed.

**Non-invasive ventilation** (NIV), on the other hand, is more commonly used in pulmonology and involves the use of nasal or facial masks that allow the patient to receive a pressurized airflow without the need for intubation. This type of ventilation is often used in pneumology departments for patients suffering from sleep apnea, acute or chronic respiratory failure, or in cases of COPD decompensation. NIV helps to reduce the work of breathing by facilitating the inflow and outflow of air from the lungs, thus improving oxygenation and carbon dioxide elimination. For the patient, this can make an immense difference, reducing the sensation of breathlessness and improving the quality of sleep and daily life. The caregiver plays a central role in supporting NIV patients, helping them adapt to the mask, monitoring ventilation comfort and efficiency, and regularly checking skin condition to prevent irritation from prolonged mask use.

**Oxygen therapy**, on the other hand, is a treatment that involves administering oxygen to a patient in order to maintain sufficient levels of oxygen in the blood. It is widely used in pulmonology, whether temporarily for patients suffering from acute respiratory infections such as pneumonia, or on a long-term basis for patients with chronic respiratory diseases such as COPD or pulmonary fibrosis. The aim of oxygen therapy is to compensate for the oxygen deficit caused by altered lungs that are no longer able to capture and exchange sufficient gas.

Oxygen therapy can be administered via several devices, depending on the patient's needs. Nasal cannulae are often used to deliver oxygen at low flow rates, enabling the patient to continue speaking and eating without hindrance. For greater needs, oxygen masks can be used, providing a higher concentration of oxygen. In some patients in acute respiratory distress, high-flow devices or oxygen tanks can be used to deliver the maximum amount of oxygen in a short space of time. In cases of prolonged home oxygen therapy, oxygen concentrators can be installed so that patients can receive a constant flow of oxygen as part of their daily routine.

The nursing auxiliary plays a major role in the management of oxygen therapy. They ensure that oxygen devices are correctly installed, check the flow rates prescribed by the doctor, and make sure that patients are comfortable with their equipment. An important aspect of monitoring also involves spotting any signs of hyperoxia (too much oxygen in the blood) or hypoxia (too little oxygen), such as headaches, confusion or cyanosis, and immediately informing the nurse or doctor. Oxygen therapy, especially long-term use, can lead to nasal dryness and skin irritation. The caregiver must therefore ensure that the nasal mucosa is hydrated, and monitor the condition of the skin around areas where the devices come into contact.

Finally, **aerosols** are another crucial tool in pulmonology, used primarily to deliver drugs directly to the lungs. This treatment is commonly used in patients with asthma, COPD or respiratory infections requiring local treatments such as bronchodilators, corticosteroids or antibiotics. Aerosols enable targeted, effective drug delivery, by transforming liquids into fine particles that the patient inhales directly into the respiratory tract.

Aerosols can be administered via nebulizers, which turn the medication into a mist that the patient breathes in, or via metered-dose inhalers, which are more portable and commonly used by asthma and COPD patients. The effectiveness of aerosols depends largely on the patient's inhalation technique. Here, the caregiver's role is to ensure that the patient uses the device correctly. This includes explaining the steps involved, such as shaking the inhaler, positioning the mouth properly around the mouthpiece, and inhaling slowly and deeply to allow the drug particles to reach the small bronchioles. If the patient uses a nebulizer, the caregiver must ensure that it is properly maintained, and that the device is clean to avoid contamination or infection.

Assisted ventilation, oxygen therapy and aerosols are essential tools in the treatment of pneumology patients. Each device has a specific function, but all share the same objective: to improve the patient's ability to breathe and exchange gases efficiently in the lungs. The role of the caregiver in managing these devices is vital, ensuring not only correct technical set-up, but also human accompaniment to help the patient understand and accept these often intimidating or uncomfortable treatments. By being attentive to the patient's needs and comfort, the caregiver contributes directly to the success of these respiratory therapies, while preserving the patient's quality of life.

   ◦   The caregiver's role in supervision and maintenance

The caregiver's role in monitoring and maintenance in pulmonology is vital to ensure the safety, comfort and well-being of patients, as well as to guarantee the effectiveness of the treatments administered. Working in close collaboration with the nurse and physician, the caregiver plays a central role in the day-to-day care of patients, monitoring their clinical condition, maintaining medical devices in good working order, and playing an active part in preventing complications. This role goes far beyond mere technical tasks, encompassing close and continuous observation of the patient's condition, as well as rigorous maintenance of equipment essential to respiratory therapy.

**Clinical monitoring** is one of the caregivers' main tasks. In pulmonology, where respiratory pathologies can progress rapidly, it's crucial to keep a close eye on patients' vital signs, and to be on the lookout for early warning signs of respiratory deterioration. The caregiver frequently assesses the patient's respiratory rate, the appearance of breathing (for example, whether there is visible intercostal indrawing or shortness of breath), and oxygen saturation using a saturometer. Signs such as cyanosis (bluish coloration of the lips or extremities), shallow or rapid breathing, or abnormal breath sounds such as wheezing, are immediate indicators that medical intervention may be required. The caregiver must then communicate these observations to the nurse or doctor, so that treatment adjustments can be made quickly.

Clinical monitoring is not limited to the observation of respiratory parameters. The caregiver also plays an important role in detecting signs of discomfort or distress in patients, often silent but indicative of underlying problems. For example, a patient who suddenly becomes agitated or has difficulty finding a comfortable position may be compensating for respiratory discomfort. Similarly, excessive fatigue, drowsiness or mental confusion may indicate hypercapnia (excess carbon dioxide in the blood) or hypoxia (oxygen deficiency), requiring immediate assessment and therapeutic adjustments. The caregiver's constant attention can anticipate and prevent emergency situations by reporting any significant change in the patient's condition.

In addition to clinical supervision, the nursing auxiliary plays an essential role in the **maintenance of medical devices**, such as oxygen therapy, assisted ventilation or aerosols. Such equipment is often vital for patients suffering from severe or chronic respiratory pathologies, and its proper functioning is essential to ensure effective treatment. Caregivers must ensure that these devices are correctly installed and adjusted according to medical prescriptions. For example, for a patient undergoing oxygen therapy, it is essential to check that the oxygen flow rate is correctly adjusted, that the nasal cannula or oxygen mask is comfortably positioned, and that the patient feels no discomfort from the equipment. The caregiver must also watch for signs of skin irritation or nasal dryness, often caused by prolonged use of these devices, and suggest solutions to alleviate these discomforts.

**Regular maintenance** of equipment is another essential aspect of the caregiver's role. Respiratory equipment, if not properly maintained, can become a source of infection or complications. For example, non-invasive ventilation masks and nebulizer tips need to be cleaned and disinfected regularly to prevent the proliferation of bacteria and fungi. The caregiver is responsible for ensuring that all devices are clean and in good working order. This involves not only daily maintenance, but also vigilance for oxygen leaks or signs of wear on the devices, which could affect the effectiveness of the treatment. In some cases, the orderly may also have to help maintain more complex equipment, such as oxygen concentrators or ventilators, in collaboration with the hospital's technical teams.

Monitoring and maintenance of **aerosol devices** are also part of the caregiver's responsibilities. In the case of aerosol treatments, used to administer drugs such as bronchodilators or corticosteroids, it is crucial to ensure that the patient is using the device correctly to guarantee effective treatment. The caregiver must ensure that the nebulizer is clean and functional, and that the patient understands how to use it. Incorrect use of these devices can reduce the effectiveness of the inhaled medication, or worse, cause further irritation of the airways. By teaching the patient the correct inhalation the ,technique caregiver contributes directly to improving therapeutic management.

Another aspect of care is the management of the patient's environment. The caregiver ensures that the patient's immediate environment is clean, well ventilated and adapted to his or her respiratory needs. Indeed, for patients suffering from chronic respiratory diseases, the quality of the ambient air is of crucial importance. The caregiver must ensure that the room is free from dust, pollutants or potential allergens that could exacerbate the patient's respiratory symptoms. Controlling air humidity, for example, can be crucial, especially for patients on long-term oxygen therapy, as overly dry air can dry out the respiratory mucosa.

Finally, the caregiver's role in monitoring and maintenance is not limited to technical aspects alone. It also includes helping patients to manage these devices. Many patients undergoing oxygen therapy or assisted ventilation at home may find it difficult to manage these devices independently. The caregiver plays the role of educator, explaining how to handle the equipment correctly, how to spot signs of malfunction, and how to adjust the devices if necessary. This support helps patients to become more autonomous, while ensuring that treatments are correctly followed.

# Chapter 2

# Anatomy and Respiratory Physiology

- **Reminder of airway anatomy**
  ○ Anatomy of the lungs, bronchi, trachea and alveoli

The anatomy of the lungs, bronchi, trachea and alveoli forms the very essence of the respiratory system, whose primary function is to enable the exchange of the gases essential to life: oxygen and carbon dioxide. This complex and remarkably organized system works in a coordinated fashion to ensure efficient and constant breathing. Understanding this anatomy is essential for understanding how the lungs and airways function, and the pathologies that can affect them.

The **trachea**, often described as the main trunk of the respiratory tree, is a rigid, flexible duct located in the lower part of the neck and upper part of the thorax. It follows the larynx, through which air enters after passing through the nose or mouth. The trachea is made up of "C"-shaped cartilage, which gives it rigidity and stability, while allowing a certain flexibility, essential for neck movements and breathing. The inside of the trachea is lined with a respiratory mucosa containing cilia and mucus-secreting cells. This system traps and evacuates inhaled particles, such as dust or micro-organisms, by pushing them outwards through coughing or secretions. At its lower end, the trachea divides into two **main bronchi**, left and right, which direct air to each lung.

The bronchi are semi-rigid ducts that continue to carry air to the lungs. From the tracheal bifurcation, each main bronchus enters its respective lung: the right bronchus goes to the right lung, and the left bronchus to the left lung. At this point, they subdivide into lobar bronchi, then into segmental bronchi, forming an increasingly fine, branched network. This branching phenomenon gives the image of a true "bronchial tree". The structure of the bronchi is similar to that of the trachea, with cartilage to maintain their opening and a ciliated inner mucosa. As the bronchi divide, they become smaller and more flexible, gradually transforming into bronchioles, which are the smallest branches of the bronchial system and no longer contain cartilage. The bronchioles distribute air throughout the lungs to the functional units of respiration: the alveoli.

The **lungs**, located in the ribcage on either side of the heart, are the main organs of respiration. Each lung is enveloped by a thin membrane called the **pleura**, which forms a double layer: a parietal pleura that lines the inside of the rib cage, and a visceral pleura that directly covers the lungs. Between these two layers lies a space called the pleural cavity, containing a small amount of fluid that allows the lungs to expand and retract as they glide frictionlessly against the chest wall during breathing. The right lung is divided into three lobes - upper, middle and lower - while the left lung, slightly smaller due to the presence of the heart, has only two - the upper and lower lobes. These lobes are themselves subdivided into segments, each corresponding to a segmental bronchus, ensuring even air distribution throughout the lung.

The lungs are responsible for gas exchange, a process that takes place in the **alveoli**. Alveoli are tiny, cluster-shaped air sacs at the ends of the bronchioles. There are several hundred million of them in each lung, providing a considerable exchange surface for oxygen and carbon dioxide. Each alveolus is surrounded by a dense network of blood capillaries, creating an ideal meeting point between inhaled air and venous blood from the heart. The walls of the alveoli are extremely thin, allowing gases to diffuse rapidly. When oxygen-rich air enters the alveoli, the oxygen passes through these walls into the capillary bloodstream, where it is transported to the body's cells. At the same time, carbon dioxide, produced by the cells and returned to the lungs via the venous blood, diffuses from the capillaries into the alveoli, to be expelled from the body during exhalation.

The architecture of the alveoli, with their immense surface area, is optimized to maximize these gas exchanges. The alveoli are lined with a thin layer of liquid, called surfactant, which plays a crucial role in reducing the surface tension of the alveolar walls. Without surfactant, the alveoli would tend to collapse, rendering breathing ineffective. Surfactant keeps the alveoli open, and helps to distribute air evenly throughout each alveolar sac, even during exhalation, when intrapulmonary pressure falls.

The anatomy of the lungs, bronchi, trachea and alveoli forms a remarkably organized system, designed to ensure fluid, continuous breathing. Each structure plays a specific and indispensable role, from the transport of air through the trachea and bronchi, to the diffusion of gases in the alveoli. This complex mechanism ensures that every cell in the body receives the oxygen it needs to function, while eliminating carbon dioxide, a by-product of cellular metabolism. Understanding this anatomy is also key to understanding various respiratory pathologies, from bronchial obstructions in asthma, to alveolar destruction in COPD, to infections affecting the lungs as in pneumonia. The proper functioning of this system is crucial to health, and any disturbance at any of these levels can have major repercussions on overall respiratory capacity.

○    Pulmonary circulation and gas exchange

**Pulmonary circulation** and **gas exchange** are essential processes in the functioning of the human body, allowing oxygenation of the blood and elimination of carbon dioxide. This complex system ensures oxygen supply to all body cells, and plays a key role in maintaining acid-base balance and metabolic functions. The efficiency of pulmonary circulation and gas exchange depends on fine coordination between the respiratory and circulatory systems.

The pulmonary circulation, also known as the **small circulation**, begins in the **right heart**. Oxygen-poor blood, loaded with carbon dioxide after having circulated throughout the body, is collected by the vena cava (superior and inferior), which discharges this blood into the heart's **right atrium**. When the right atrium contracts, the blood flows into the **right ventricle**, which in turn contracts to propel the blood to the **pulmonary arteries**. Unlike the body's other arteries, which carry oxygenated blood, the pulmonary arteries carry deoxygenated blood to the lungs. They branch out in an ever finer network to supply each lobe, segment and finally each alveolus of the lung.

Once inside the lungs, the pulmonary arteries continue to divide into smaller vessels, called **capillaries**, which surround each pulmonary **alveolus**. The alveoli are the functional units of the lungs where **gas exchange** takes place. This vital process oxygenates the blood and eliminates carbon dioxide. The walls of the alveoli and capillaries are extremely thin, allowing gases to pass easily from the air in the alveoli to the blood, and vice versa.

**Gas exchange** itself takes place via a process of passive diffusion. Oxygen in the inspired air reaches the alveoli, where it passes through the thin alveolar wall into the surrounding pulmonary capillaries. Once in the bloodstream, oxygen binds primarily to **hemoglobin**, a protein found in red blood cells, which transports it to all the body's cells. This process is guided by a concentration gradient: oxygen diffuses from areas of higher concentration (in the alveoli) to those of lower concentration (in the blood).

At the same time, the **carbon dioxide** present in the venous blood is expelled from the capillaries into the alveoli. This gas is a by-product of cellular metabolism, which must be eliminated to prevent blood acidification. Here again, diffusion occurs as a function of the concentration gradient: carbon dioxide moves from the capillaries, where its concentration is higher, to the alveoli, where it is lower. This process removes carbon dioxide from the body during exhalation.

So, with each respiratory cycle, inhaled air brings oxygen to the alveoli, while carbon dioxide is expelled during exhalation. This process is extremely efficient, thanks to the immense exchange surface provided by the lungs' millions of alveoli. Together, these alveoli provide an estimated 70 to 100 square meters of surface area - comparable to the surface of a tennis court - and ensure rapid, efficient oxygenation of the blood.

Once gas exchange is complete, the now oxygen-rich blood is collected by the **pulmonary veins**. Unlike the pulmonary arteries, which carry deoxygenated blood, the pulmonary veins carry oxygenated blood from the lungs back to the **left heart**, to the **left atrium**. From there, the blood passes into the **left ventricle**, which, when it contracts, propels this oxygenated blood into the **aorta**. The blood is then distributed throughout the body via the **large circulation** system to supply organs and tissues with oxygen, ensuring the body's proper functioning.

The efficiency of pulmonary circulation and gas exchange depends on a number of factors. One of the most important is lung **ventilation**, i.e. the ability to bring oxygen-rich air into the alveoli and expel carbon dioxide-laden air. Pathologies such as COPD or asthma can compromise this ventilation by reducing the flow of air to the alveoli. This causes an imbalance between oxygen supply and the body's needs, leading to symptoms of dyspnea and hypoxia.

Another determining factor is **pulmonary perfusion**, i.e. the ability of the pulmonary blood vessels to carry blood to the alveoli for gas exchange. Certain diseases, such as pulmonary embolism, can obstruct blood vessels in the lungs, blocking perfusion to part of the alveoli and preventing blood oxygenation in these areas. This type of disturbance can lead to hypoxemia, i.e. a reduction in the concentration of oxygen in the blood, with potentially serious consequences for vital organs.

Proper gas exchange also depends on the integrity of the alveolar membranes. In certain pathologies, such as **pulmonary fibrosis**, thickening of the alveolar-capillary membrane makes gas diffusion more difficult, slowing down blood oxygenation and carbon dioxide elimination. In addition, infection or inflammation of the lungs, as in pneumonia, can fill the alveoli with fluid or pus, blocking gas exchange and causing respiratory distress.

- **Normal functioning of the respiratory system**
  ○ Breathing processes: inhalation and exhalation

The breathing process, which includes **inhalation** and **exhalation**, is a vital phenomenon by which the human body exchanges gases with the environment. This mechanism ensures the supply of oxygen necessary for cellular life and the elimination of carbon dioxide, the product of metabolism. This process is automatic, regulated by the nervous system and constantly adapted to the body's needs, whether at rest or during physical exertion. Breathing, though natural and automatic, relies on fine coordination between the respiratory muscles, the lungs and the central nervous system.

**Inspiration** is the first phase of the respiratory cycle, when air is drawn from the upper airways into the lungs. This process begins with contraction of the **diaphragm**, a large, dome-shaped muscle that separates the thoracic cavity from the abdominal cavity. As the diaphragm contracts, it lowers, increasing the volume of the thoracic cavity. At the same time, the **external intercostal muscles** between the ribs also contract, lifting the ribs outwards and further increasing the volume of the thoracic cavity. This thoracic expansion causes a drop in pressure inside the lungs, creating a negative pressure relative to the surrounding air. As gases always move from high-pressure to low-pressure zones, outside air is drawn into the lungs through the trachea, bronchi and bronchioles to the alveoli.

In the **alveoli**, the **gas exchange** process takes place. The oxygen contained in the inspired air passes through the thin walls of the alveoli into the blood capillaries, where it binds with the hemoglobin present in the red blood cells. At the same time, carbon dioxide, produced by the body's cells and transported to the lungs by venous blood, diffuses from the capillaries to the alveoli, where it is eliminated during exhalation. This process takes place quickly and efficiently, thanks to the huge surface area of the alveoli and the close proximity of the pulmonary capillaries.

45

Once inhalation has filled the lungs with fresh air and gas exchange has taken place, the body must rid itself of accumulated carbon dioxide. This is when **exhalation** begins, the phase when air is expelled from the lungs. Unlike inspiration, expiration is a **passive** process at rest. It occurs when the inspiratory muscles relax: the diaphragm returns to its original position, the external intercostal muscles relax and the thoracic cage returns to its resting volume. This relaxation reduces the volume of the thoracic cavity, increasing the pressure inside the lungs. This pressure then becomes higher than atmospheric pressure, naturally pushing air out of the lungs via the respiratory tract, the trachea and finally the nasal or oral passages.

During exhalation, the carbon dioxide that has accumulated in the alveoli after gas exchange is expelled with the exhaled air. As a result, exhaled air contains a higher concentration of carbon dioxide and less oxygen than inhaled air.

Exhalation is a passive act under normal conditions, but it can become **active** in certain situations, such as during physical exertion or when the body needs to evacuate air more quickly. In this case, other muscles intervene to force expiration. The **internal intercostal muscles**, for example, contract to lower the ribs and further reduce the volume of the rib cage. Similarly, the **abdominal muscles** may contract to increase pressure on the diaphragm, helping to expel air more quickly and efficiently. This mechanism is particularly important when coughing, which is a forced exhalation designed to clear the airways.

The breathing process is controlled by the **respiratory center**, located in the brain stem, more precisely in the medulla oblongata. This nerve center automatically regulates the frequency and depth of breathing in response to the body's need for oxygen and variations in blood carbon dioxide levels. Chemoreceptors, located in the aorta and carotid arteries, constantly monitor oxygen, carbon dioxide and blood pH levels. When carbon dioxide accumulates in the blood, the chemoreceptors send signals to the respiratory center to increase the frequency and depth of breathing. Conversely, if carbon dioxide levels drop too low, the respiratory center slows down breathing.

Breathing regulation is therefore largely **involuntary**, but it can also be influenced by voluntary or emotional factors. For example, we can voluntarily control our breathing by slowing it down, as in a relaxation practice, or by speeding it up, as in intense physical exercise. Similarly, strong emotions such as fear or anxiety can cause breathing to accelerate, known as **hyperventilation**.

Breathing may seem like a simple, automatic process, but it's actually a complex, finely-tuned phenomenon. The harmonious interplay between inhalation, which brings oxygen to the body's cells, and exhalation, which removes carbon dioxide, is crucial to maintaining the body's homeostasis and ensuring its proper functioning. Any disruption to this mechanism, whether caused by airway obstruction, muscle weakness or damage to the lungs themselves, can lead to serious respiratory disorders. In the management of respiratory pathologies, one of the main objectives is to restore or support this breathing process to ensure optimal gas exchange and patient survival.

   ◦   Oxygen and carbon dioxide transport
The **transport of oxygen** and **carbon dioxide** in the human body is an essential process for maintaining homeostasis and cell function. This transport is carried out mainly by the blood system, which links the lungs, where gas exchange takes place, to the body's tissues, which use oxygen to produce energy and eliminate carbon dioxide as a metabolic waste product. This continuous double transport is finely orchestrated by complex physiological mechanisms involving red blood cells and the chemical properties of gases.

Once inhaled into the lungs, **oxygen** reaches the **alveoli**, where it diffuses through the thin alveolar-capillary membrane into the pulmonary capillaries. Once in the blood, oxygen binds primarily to **hemoglobin**, a protein found in **red blood cells** (erythrocytes). Hemoglobin has the ability to bind oxygen reversibly, thanks to its four iron-containing binding sites. This affinity for oxygen enables hemoglobin to capture up to four oxygen molecules per hemoglobin molecule. Around 98% of oxygen in the blood is transported in this way, the remainder being dissolved directly in blood plasma.

Once bound to hemoglobin, oxygen is transported by the **circulatory system** to the body's various tissues and organs. Oxygenated blood from the lungs is pumped by the **left heart** into the systemic circulation. When it reaches the tissue capillaries, oxygen is released from the hemoglobin in response to the metabolic demands of the cells. This process is aided by a concentration gradient: oxygen naturally moves from areas of high concentration (the blood) to areas of low concentration (the cells). This mechanism is amplified by local tissue conditions, such as acidification linked to increased metabolic activity, and increased temperature, which reduce the affinity of hemoglobin for oxygen, thus facilitating its release.

Once released, oxygen enters the cells where it is used in the **mitochondria** for the process of cellular respiration, a mechanism that produces the energy needed by the cell in the form of **ATP** (adenosine triphosphate). This process, in turn, generates **carbon dioxide** ($CO_2$) as a waste product.

**Carbon dioxide**, produced by cells, must be eliminated from the body to maintain acid-base balance and avoid the accumulation of acids in tissues, which could lead to cellular dysfunction. $CO_2$ diffuses from cells into the blood capillaries, where it is transported in several forms. Around 7% of carbon dioxide is dissolved directly in blood plasma, but the majority is transported as **bicarbonate** ($HCO_3$-), the result of a chemical reaction between $CO_2$ and water ($H_2O$) in red blood cells, catalyzed by an enzyme called **carbonic anhydrase**. This process converts carbon dioxide into bicarbonate, a soluble and easily transportable form in plasma.

Another fraction of $CO_2$ (around 23%) binds directly to hemoglobin proteins, forming a compound called **carbamate**. Unlike oxygen, which binds to the iron sites of hemoglobin, $CO_2$ binds to other sites on the molecule. Moreover, hemoglobin, in its deoxygenated form, has a higher affinity for carbon dioxide, which favors its transport from tissues to the lungs, where $CO_2$ can be eliminated.

When venous blood, rich in carbon dioxide, returns to the **lungs** via the right heart and pulmonary circulation, the reverse process occurs. Dissolved carbon dioxide in the form of bicarbonate is converted back into $CO_2$ in the red blood cells, and then diffuses across the alveolar-capillary membrane to be evacuated into the alveoli. Exhalation then releases this carbon dioxide into the surrounding air. This cycle is constant and essential for maintaining a stable level of $CO_2$ in the blood, thus avoiding **acidosis** (excessive accumulation of acid in the blood) or **alkalosis** (excessive depletion of acids), two imbalances that can have serious consequences for the body.

The **regulation of this gas transport** is finely controlled by the **respiratory center** located in the brain stem, more precisely in the medulla oblongata. This center receives information from **chemoreceptors** located in the aorta and carotid arteries, which constantly monitor oxygen and carbon dioxide levels in the blood. If $CO_2$ levels rise (such as during exercise or in cases of hypoventilation), the respiratory center increases the frequency and depth of breathing to remove more $CO_2$ and increase oxygen intake. Conversely, if $CO_2$ levels are too low, breathing is slowed to maintain equilibrium.

This process of transporting oxygen and carbon dioxide is essential to life. Oxygen, captured in the lungs, is transported by hemoglobin to supply every cell in the body, while carbon dioxide, produced by these same cells, is returned to the lungs for elimination. This double transport, ensured by the circulatory system, is a remarkable example of the human body's efficiency in maintaining internal equilibrium (homeostasis), even in the face of changing needs, such as during physical exertion or in varied environmental conditions. Any disruption to this process, whether due to respiratory or cardiovascular disease or hemoglobin dysfunction, can lead to serious disorders, underlining the crucial importance of these mechanisms for the survival and health of the organism.

- **Common respiratory pathologies in pneumology**
  - COPD, asthma, emphysema, chronic bronchitis

**COPD**, **asthma**, **emphysema** and **chronic bronchitis** are respiratory diseases that affect the airways and lungs, causing progressive impairment of breathing. Although these diseases share common features, they differ in their mechanisms, causes and management. Understanding these diseases is essential to providing appropriate care for patients suffering from them, as they can have a profound impact on quality of life.

## Chronic Obstructive Pulmonary Disease (COPD)

**COPD**, or **chronic obstructive pulmonary disease**, is a chronic respiratory illness characterized by persistent airway obstruction that restricts airflow to the lungs. This obstruction is generally progressive and irreversible. COPD comprises two main conditions: **emphysema** and **chronic bronchitis**, which often coexist in patients. It is mainly caused by exposure to long-term irritants, particularly tobacco smoke, but also by air pollution and occupational exposure to dusts and chemicals.

In COPD, the combination of bronchial inflammation (chronic bronchitis) and alveolar destruction (emphysema) reduces the lungs' ability to exchange gases efficiently. COPD patients often experience **dyspnea** (shortness of breath), **chronic cough** and excessive mucus production. These symptoms are often insidious, progressing slowly over the years. As the disease progresses, airflow limitation worsens, causing respiratory distress even during minor daily activities.

The diagnosis of COPD is confirmed by lung function tests, including **spirometry**, which measures lung capacity and the rate at which air is exhaled. Treatment for COPD includes bronchodilator drugs to open up the airways, inhaled corticosteroids to reduce inflammation, and respiratory rehabilitation programs. In more severe cases, **oxygen therapy** or **assisted ventilation** may be necessary.

## Asthma

**Asthma** is another chronic respiratory disease, characterized by recurrent inflammation of the bronchial tubes leading to **bronchial hyperreactivity**, i.e. a tendency of the airways to constrict in response to various stimuli, such as allergens, infections, exercise or irritants. This bronchial constriction is reversible, which distinguishes asthma from COPD, where obstruction is progressive and irreversible.

Patients with asthma experience attacks marked by **wheezing**, chest tightness, **coughing** and difficulty breathing, which can occur unpredictably. Asthma attacks can range in severity from mild discomfort to severe, life-threatening respiratory distress. These attacks are triggered by factors such as dust, pollen, smoke, exercise or respiratory infections.

Asthma treatment relies on fast-acting bronchodilators, such as **beta-agonists**, for immediate relief of symptoms during an attack, and background medications, such as **inhaled corticosteroids**, to control chronic inflammation and prevent attacks. Unlike COPD, asthma patients can improve their symptoms with appropriate treatment, and their respiratory function can be relatively normal between attacks.

## Emphysema

**Emphysema** is one of the two main components of COPD. It is characterized by the **progressive destruction of the alveoli**, the small air sacs at the end of the bronchioles, where gas exchange takes place. This destruction leads to a loss of elasticity in the lungs, reducing their capacity to expel air efficiently. As a result, emphysema patients have difficulty emptying their lungs completely during exhalation, leading to air accumulation in the lungs and a sensation of shortness of breath, even at rest.

Smoking is the main cause of emphysema, as the toxic substances in cigarette smoke cause chronic inflammation of the airways and irreversible damage to the alveoli. As the disease progresses, patients can suffer from extreme fatigue, muscle weakness and disabling dyspnea, making even light activities difficult to perform.

Treatment of emphysema, like that of COPD, relies mainly on bronchodilators, corticosteroids and respiratory rehabilitation. In some advanced cases, surgery may be considered to remove the most affected areas of the lung, or a **lung transplant** may be necessary in severely affected patients.

## Chronic bronchitis

**Chronic bronchitis**, another component of COPD, is defined by a persistent **productive cough**, with mucus **expectoration**, lasting at least three months a year for two consecutive years. It is caused by inflammation of the bronchial tubes, leading to excessive mucus production and narrowing of the airways, making breathing difficult. As with emphysema, smoking is the main risk factor for chronic bronchitis, but air pollution and exposure to chemical irritants also play a role.

Patients with chronic bronchitis often experience frequent lung infections, as excess mucus and damaged bronchial tubes provide a breeding ground for bacteria. Symptoms include a persistent cough, shortness of breath and general fatigue. Unlike asthma, where symptoms may be intermittent and reversible, chronic bronchitis causes progressive and permanent deterioration of the bronchial tubes.

Treatment of chronic bronchitis aims to reduce symptoms and prevent exacerbations. It includes bronchodilators, corticosteroids and antibiotics in case of infection. Smoking cessation is the most effective measure for slowing the progression of the disease.

　　　　　○　　Respiratory infections: pneumonia, tuberculosis, pleurisy

**Respiratory infections**, such as **pneumonia, tuberculosis** and **pleurisy**, are diseases that affect the lungs and adjacent structures of the respiratory system. These infections, whether bacterial, viral or fungal, can vary in severity, from mild infections to life-threatening conditions. Each of these infections has different clinical features and pathological mechanisms, requiring specific diagnostic and therapeutic approaches. However, they all share a common ability to cause inflammation of the lungs and impairment of respiratory function, which can lead to serious complications if not treated appropriately.

# Pneumonia

**Pneumonia** is an acute lung infection that leads to inflammation of the alveoli, the small air sacs where gas exchange takes place. In pneumonia, these alveoli fill with fluid, pus or cellular debris, disrupting respiratory function and making it difficult to oxygenate the blood adequately. Pneumonia can be caused by a variety of pathogens, including bacteria (such as **Streptococcus**

**pneumoniae**, the most common cause), viruses (including respiratory viruses such as influenza), and in some cases, fungi. It can affect one or more lobes of the lung, and its forms can vary from mild to severe pneumonia, often accompanied by complications.

Typical symptoms of pneumonia include high **fever**, **chills**, **productive cough** with purulent sputum, chest pain and **dyspnea** (shortness of breath). In severe cases, especially in the elderly or immunocompromised, pneumonia can lead to respiratory failure, requiring hospitalization or even intensive care.

Diagnosis of pneumonia is based on clinical examination, which may reveal **crackles** or abnormal breath sounds when the lungs are auscultated, as well as complementary tests such as **chest x-rays**, which show opacities or infiltrates in infected areas of the lungs. Microbiological analyses, such as **blood cultures** or **sputum cultures**, can be performed to identify the causative pathogen and adjust treatment.

Treatment of pneumonia depends on the causative agent. Bacterial pneumonia requires **antibiotics**, usually administered orally for moderate forms, or intravenously for more severe infections. Viral forms may require antivirals, although treatment is often symptomatic. Good hydration, cough suppressants and sometimes oxygen therapy are used to relieve symptoms. In at-risk patients (elderly, immunocompromised), prevention through vaccination (particularly against pneumococcus and influenza) is key to reducing the incidence of pneumonia.

## Tuberculosis

**Tuberculosis** is a chronic lung infection caused by the bacterium **Mycobacterium tuberculosis**, which is transmitted by air, mainly via droplets coughed or sneezed up by an infected person. Although tuberculosis can affect other organs, such as the bones, kidneys or brain, it mainly affects the lungs, where it causes chronic and progressive damage if left untreated. Tuberculosis remains a major public health problem, particularly in developing countries, although cases have also increased in certain at-risk populations in industrialized countries (notably the immunocompromised or people living in precarious conditions).

**Pulmonary tuberculosis** often manifests itself as a **persistent cough** lasting more than three weeks, sometimes accompanied by **bloody sputum** (hemoptysis), **low-grade fever**, **night sweats** and **progressive weight loss**. The clinical picture is often insidious, evolving slowly, and diagnosis may be delayed. The infection may remain latent for years without causing symptoms, and it is only when it reactivates, often due to a weakening of the immune system, that it becomes symptomatic.

Diagnosis is based on **tuberculin tests** (such as the Mantoux test), **chest X-rays** and bacteriological analyses (sputum culture, PCR to detect the genetic material of the tubercle bacillus). Tuberculosis treatment is lengthy and relies on a combination of several **specific** antibiotics, including isoniazid, rifampicin, ethambutol and pyrazinamide. This treatment, known as **multidrug antituberculosis therapy**, must be followed for at least six months to ensure complete elimination of the bacillus and avoid the emergence of drug resistance. Prevention is based on **BCG** vaccination in countries where the disease is endemic, and early detection and treatment of latent cases.

## Pleuresis

**Pleurisy** is an inflammation of the **pleura**, the double membrane that surrounds the lungs and lines the inside of the rib cage. The pleura is normally lubricated by a thin layer of fluid, allowing the lungs to expand and contract without friction during breathing. When inflammation affects the pleura, it causes acute chest pain, often described as **throbbing** or **stinging**, which is exacerbated by deep breathing, coughing or movement. Pleurisy can be caused by infection (viral, bacterial or fungal), underlying conditions such as pneumonia or tuberculosis, or autoimmune diseases such as lupus.

Pleurisy is sometimes accompanied by **pleural effusion**, i.e. an accumulation of fluid in the pleural space, which can compress the lungs and aggravate breathing difficulty. Depending on the nature of the accumulated fluid (transudate or exudate), this may give clues to the underlying cause of pleural inflammation. For example, a purulent pleural effusion (purulent pleurisy) suggests a bacterial infection, while a clear effusion is often associated with heart or liver disease.

Diagnosis of pleurisy is based on clinical examination (auscultation revealing pleural friction), **thoracic X-rays** or **ultrasound**, and sometimes **thoracentesis**, which involves removing pleural fluid for analysis. Treatment of pleurisy depends on the underlying cause. If infection is the cause, antibiotics are used, while **anti-inflammatories** and **analgesics** are prescribed to relieve pain. In cases of significant pleural effusion, evacuation of the fluid may be necessary to enable the patient to breathe more easily.

         ○    Interstitial diseases and pulmonary fibrosis

**Interstitial diseases** and **pulmonary fibrosis** are chronic respiratory conditions that affect the pulmonary **interstitium**, the thin layer of tissue between the pulmonary alveoli and blood capillaries, where gas exchange takes place. These diseases are often grouped together under the term **diffuse interstitial lung disease** (DIP) and are characterized by inflammation and progressive scarring of the interstitium, leading to a loss of elasticity in the lungs and a reduction in their ability to function properly. The process of fibrosecorresponds to the thickening and rigidification of lung tissue, caused by an excess of scar tissue. This limits the lungs' capacity to expand and exchange gases, leading to progressive respiratory failure.

# Interstitial diseases

**Interstitial lung diseases** encompass a wide range of conditions affecting the interstitium of the lungs. The term includes dozens of conditions, some of which are idiopathic (with no known cause), while others are secondary to environmental exposures, autoimmune diseases, infections or drugs. These include conditions such as **sarcoidosis, hypersensitivity pneumonitis** and **idiopathic interstitial lung disease** (ILD).

In interstitial disease, the initial inflammation of the interstitium can gradually lead to fibrosis. The interstitium becomes thicker and stiffer, making it difficult for the lungs to expand with each inspiration. Inflammation and fibrosis also disrupt **gas exchange** in the alveoli, reducing blood oxygenation. Patients suffering from these diseases often present symptoms of **dyspnea** (shortness of breath), which worsens over time, especially on exertion. Other symptoms may include a persistent **dry cough**, fatigue, and in advanced stages, **digital hippocratism** (deformed nails and fingers).

Interstitial diseases can have a variety of origins. They can be caused by chronic environmental exposures, such as inhalation of organic or inorganic particles (e.g. silica dust, asbestos or mold). These exposures can lead to pathologies such as **silicosis** or **asbestosis**. Other interstitial diseases are **autoimmune** in origin, as in the case of **rheumatoid arthritis, scleroderma** or **systemic lupus erythematosus**, where the immune system attacks lung tissue, causing inflammation and damage. Finally, certain medications used over the long term, such as certain cancer treatments, antibiotics or anti-inflammatories, can also induce interstitial lesions.

## Idiopathic pulmonary fibrosis

**Idiopathic pulmonary fibrosis** (IPF) is one of the most severe and frequent forms of interstitial disease. It is a progressive condition in which lung tissue becomes increasingly rigid and fibrous, without any precise cause being identified. The term "idiopathic" means that the origin of this fibrosis is unknown, although it is likely that genetic and environmental factors, as well as immune abnormalities, play a role.

In IPF, the pulmonary interstitium is progressively invaded by **scar tissue**, a phenomenon known as **fibrosis**. This scar tissue makes the lungs rigid and hampers their ability to expand properly, reducing their respiratory function. As a result, IPF patients experience increasing shortness of breath on exertion, and even at rest in more advanced stages. They may also suffer from a dry, persistent cough, weight loss and fatigue. Idiopathic pulmonary fibrosis is an incurable disease, and its course is often unpredictable, although most patients experience progressive deterioration.

Diagnosis of IPF is based on several tests, including **high-resolution thoracic computed tomography** (HR CT), which visualizes characteristic abnormalities, such as the "honeycomb" appearance of the lungs, reflecting destruction and fibrosis of lung tissue. **Respiratory function** tests generally reveal a reduction in total lung capacity, typical of restrictive diseases, and a decrease in gas diffusion.

Treatment of IPF remains limited. **Antifibrotic drugs** (such as pirfenidone and ninedanib) can slow the progression of fibrosis, but cannot cure it. **Corticosteroids** or other immunosuppressants can be used in some cases to reduce inflammation, although their efficacy is limited in pure IPF. **Respiratory rehabilitation** programs are also important to help patients maintain their quality of life by improving exercise tolerance and teaching them to manage their breath. In the terminal phase, **lung transplantation** may be considered in some patients, although this option is not always feasible due to disease progression or the patient's general condition.

# Consequences for respiratory function

**Pulmonary fibrosis**, whether idiopathic or secondary to other interstitial diseases, has major consequences for respiratory function. As lung tissue thickens and becomes rigid, the lungs lose their natural **elasticity**, making inspiration difficult. The resulting phenomenon of **pulmonary restriction** translates into a reduction in total lung capacity. At the same time, damage to the alveoli disrupts gas exchange, in particular the lungs' ability to oxygenate the blood properly and eliminate carbon dioxide. This leads to hypoxemia (reduced oxygen levels in the blood), which can worsen with effort, and even at rest in advanced stages.

Patients suffering from pulmonary fibrosis often develop **chronic respiratory failure**, sometimes requiring home oxygen therapy. Progressive dyspnea leads to a reduced ability to carry out daily activities, severely impacting patients' quality of life. In advanced cases, respiratory insufficiency can lead to cardiac complications, such as **pulmonary hypertension**, due to increased pressure in the blood vessels of the lungs, putting excessive strain on the heart.

# Chapter 3

# Welcoming patients to the Respiratory Department

- **The importance of a caring approach**
  - Creating a relationship of trust from the moment of admission

Establishing a **relationship of trust right from the time of admission** is an essential step in patient care, particularly in respiratory medicine, where respiratory ailments can give rise to considerable anxiety. From the very first contact, this relationship plays a decisive role in ensuring that care runs smoothly, that patients adhere to treatment and that their overall well-being is enhanced. Admission is often a stressful time for patients, who find themselves in a medicalized environment that is sometimes unfamiliar and worrying. It is therefore crucial that the care team, and particularly the nursing auxiliary, adopt a caring, reassuring and professional approach at this key moment.

When a patient arrives in our service, the first impression is fundamental. The **first visual and** verbal **contact** immediately **sets** the tone for the relationship. A warm welcome, with a smile, simple words and a calm tone, helps to break the initial tension. The caregiver, who is often the first to interact with the patient, plays a key role here. By clearly introducing himself and explaining his role, the caregiver demonstrates from the outset his availability and commitment to accompanying the patient. This simple approach allows the patient to feel that he or she is not a stranger in a hospital system often perceived as impersonal, but that he or she is the focus of the caregivers' attention.

**Active listening is** another key to building trust from the moment of admission. Patients, whether in respiratory distress or not, often arrive with questions, concerns and even fears about their illness or the care they are about to receive. Taking the time to listen, to let them express their fears and needs, without judgment or haste, is a sign of respect and empathy. The caregiver must be attentive not only to words, but also to the patient's non-verbal signals, such as his or her gaze, posture or breathing, which can reveal deeper anxieties. A simple phrase such as "I'm here to help you, so don't hesitate to tell me what's worrying you" can be enough to open up a space for dialogue, which is essential if the patient is to feel secure.

Information also plays a key role in creating this relationship of trust. On admission, patients may feel lost when faced with medical procedures or the use of technical equipment such as oxygen therapy or assisted ventilation. As well as carrying out the first technical steps, such as positioning the patient or taking vital signs, the nursing auxiliary must take care to **explain** each stage clearly and simply. For example, explaining why oxygen saturation needs to be monitored regularly, or what a saturometer is used for, helps to make the use of these devices less dramatic, and enables the patient to play an active role in his or her own care. This sharing of information, without excessive medical jargon, reassures the patient, who better understands what is happening to him and what the team is doing for him.

Caregivers must also **respect** the patient's **privacy and dignity**. During body care, such as bathing or getting into bed, it is important to preserve the patient's privacy as much as possible. By closing the curtains or the bedroom door, and explaining each gesture before doing so, the caregiver shows respect for the whole person, not just the patient. This attention to dignity is a fundamental element in creating a climate of trust, because it makes the patient feel respected in his or her humanity, which reduces feelings of vulnerability.

Admission is also a time when patients often need reassurance about the team that will be looking after them. The nursing auxiliary can play a **mediating** role by introducing the rest of the medical team - nurses, doctors, physiotherapists - and explaining the roles of each. This enables the patient to know who to contact for each specific need, creating a dynamic of trust and transparency between the patient and all the staff. When patients understand who is responsible for what, they can more easily get involved in their own care, and feel surrounded by a competent, supportive team.

Finally, it's important to **personalize your welcome**. Each patient has a different history, experiences and expectations. Caregivers must take these factors into account to adapt their approach. For example, a patient suffering from chronic respiratory illnesses such as COPD will often already be familiar with treatments and equipment, but may also feel a great deal of psychological fatigue linked to repeated hospitalizations. In this case, the caregiver can offer more emotional support, while respecting the patient's knowledge and experience. Conversely, a patient in hospital for the first time may be totally disorientated and need a more detailed explanation of care and how the ward works.

　　　　　　∘　　Initial questions and comments

The **first questions and observations made** when a patient is admitted to a pneumology unit are crucial to assessing the patient's state of health, and guiding the patient's care in a personalized and efficient manner. These first steps enable the care team to gather essential information on the patient's clinical condition, medical history and immediate needs. This process, although technical, must be carried out in a climate of caring and listening, in order to reassure the patient while gathering precise data to guide therapeutic decisions.

The first questions we ask patients are designed to establish an **initial assessment** of their respiratory and general condition. They enable us to identify the symptoms that led to the patient's hospitalization or consultation. One of the first important questions is: "How long have you been experiencing respiratory discomfort?" or "How long have you had difficulty breathing?" This question helps to pinpoint the onset of the problem and to understand the evolution of symptoms. Recent respiratory discomfort may point to an acute infection, such as pneumonia, while long-term discomfort could suggest a chronic disease such as COPD or pulmonary fibrosis.

Other questions follow to refine the assessment of respiratory symptoms, such as, "Do you have a cough?" "Is this cough dry or productive?" If the cough is productive, the caregiver or nurse may be interested in the nature of the **sputum**: "What is the color of the sputum? Is there any blood?" The presence of **purulent sputum** (yellow or green) may indicate a lung infection, while **bloody sputum** (hemoptysis) may suggest more serious pathologies, such as tuberculosis, pulmonary embolism or bronchial cancer. The **frequency and severity of the cough** are also important to assess, as a persistent cough, especially at night, can have a significant impact on the patient's quality of life.

**Dyspnea**, or breathlessness, is often one of the main symptoms in pneumology. It's important to assess its intensity and triggers. "Are you short of breath at rest or only on exertion?" "At what time of day do you feel the most discomfort?" "Are you able to climb stairs or walk short distances without stopping?" These questions help to measure the degree of **functional limitation** and the impact of dyspnea on the patient's daily life. If dyspnea occurs at night or while lying down, this may point to heart disease or pulmonary edema.

Questions about the patient's **medical history** and **risk factors** are also crucial in guiding the diagnosis. "Are you a smoker?" is an unavoidable question, as smoking is the most important risk factor in diseases such as COPD, emphysema or bronchial cancer. "Have you been exposed to toxic substances or dust in the course of your work?" This question is used to detect **occupational exposure** to pathogens such as asbestos, silica or other chemicals likely to cause interstitial lung disease. In addition, questioning about underlying **chronic illnesses** such as asthma, allergies or autoimmune diseases (such as rheumatoid arthritis or scleroderma) is essential for adapting management and identifying any interactions with current treatments.

Beyond the questions, the first **clinical observations** are crucial. These observations provide objective information on the patient's state of health and detect visible signs of respiratory distress. The caregiver, in collaboration with the nurse or doctor, **monitors vital signs**, taking temperature, heart rate, blood pressure and, above all, **oxygen saturation** (SpO2) using a saturometer. Saturations below 90% may indicate hypoxia, requiring immediate intervention, such as oxygen therapy.

Observation of **breathing** is also essential. The rhythm and depth of breathing can already give clues to the patient's condition. Rapid, shallow breathing may indicate **tachypnea**, often associated with respiratory distress, while a patient with **bradypnea** (slow breathing) or irregular breathing may signal more severe damage to the respiratory centers. The patient's position can also be revealing. A patient in a seated or crouched position, seeking support to breathe (the so-called tripod position), shows signs of **respiratory distress**.

**Visible signs of cyanosis**, i.e. a bluish tinge to the lips, fingers or earlobes, should be noted immediately. Cyanosis indicates severe hypoxemia, or poor oxygenation of the blood. In addition, observation of the skin, nails and extremities may reveal other clues, such as **digital hippocratism**, characterized by swelling of the last phalanges of the fingers and deformation of the nails, a sign often associated with chronic lung diseases such as pulmonary fibrosis or bronchial cancer.

Listening for **respiratory sounds** such as **crackles**, **sibilance** or **rales** during auscultation by the physician complements these initial observations. These sounds can point towards a precise diagnosis: crackles often suggest the presence of fluid in the alveoli, as in pneumonia or pulmonary fibrosis, while sibilance (wheezing) is typical of asthma or COPD.

- **Assessment of the patient's clinical condition**
  - Signs of respiratory distress (cyanosis, draught, polypnoea)

**Signs of respiratory distress**, such as **cyanosis**, **draft** and **polypnoea**, are key clinical indicators of respiratory failure or decompensation in a patient. They signal that the body is no longer able to maintain adequate gas exchange, leading to a critical drop in blood oxygenation or an inability to properly eliminate carbon dioxide. These signs need to be recognized quickly by the health-care team, as they may reveal a potentially serious situation requiring immediate intervention. Monitoring these manifestations is crucial, particularly in pneumology, where chronic or acute respiratory illnesses can suddenly become complicated.

## Cyanosis

**Cyanosis** is one of the most visible signs of respiratory distress. It manifests as a **bluish** discoloration of the skin, lips, nails or extremities, and results from a significant drop in blood oxygenation. More precisely, cyanosis occurs when the level of **deoxygenated hemoglobin** )hemoglobin that does not carry oxygen) in capillary blood exceeds a certain threshold. This reflects **hypoxemia**, i.e. a lack of oxygen in the blood. Patients with cyanosis may have bluish lips, earlobes, fingers or toes, indicating that tissues are not receiving sufficient oxygen.

Cyanosis may be **central** or **peripheral**. **Central** cyanosis occurs mainly in the lips, tongue and face, and is due to generalized hypoxemia, often as a result of severe respiratory failure. It can occur in conditions such as **acute pulmonary edema, severe pneumonia**, or an **exacerbation of COPD. Peripheral** cyanosis, on the other hand, mainly affects the extremities (hands, feet) and is linked to poor peripheral circulation or vasoconstriction of small blood vessels, as in shock or hypothermia.

When cyanosis is detected, it's crucial to act quickly to restore proper oxygenation. This may involve **oxygen therapy**, respiratory assistance or even more invasive intervention in the case of advanced respiratory failure.

# Drawing

**Drawing** is another clinical sign of respiratory distress, observed when the accessory respiratory muscles are excessively solicited in an attempt to compensate for difficulty in breathing. Normally, breathing is carried out by the **diaphragm** and **intercostal muscles**, but in the event of respiratory distress, the body mobilizes other muscles, notably in the neck, shoulders and abdomen, to aid inspiration.

Draught manifests itself as **abnormal retraction of** the intercostal spaces (between the ribs), the supra-clavicular fossae (above the clavicle), and sometimes at the base of the neck or the sternum. These visible indentations in the skin with each inhalation indicate that the patient is making an intense effort to push air into the lungs. This phenomenon is particularly common in children and infants, but can also be observed in adults in acute respiratory distress.

Draught is often associated with obstructive pathologies such as **severe asthma**, where the bronchi are narrowed, making inspiration difficult, or in conditions such as **pneumonia**, **pulmonary edema**, or **emphysema**, where the lungs' ability to inflate is compromised. This clinical sign is an important indicator of respiratory muscle exhaustion, and requires rapid intervention to relieve respiratory effort and avoid **respiratory failure**.

# Polypnea

**Polypnoea** refers to an **abnormal increase in respiratory rate**, i.e. a higher-than-normal number of breaths per minute. In a healthy adult, the normal respiratory rate is between 12 and 20 breaths per minute. When it exceeds these values, we speak of polypnoea. This phenomenon reflects the body's attempt to compensate for respiratory insufficiency by increasing ventilation to bring in more oxygen and expel more carbon dioxide.

Polypnoea is a sign of respiratory distress that can be observed in many clinical situations, such as **pneumonia**, **pulmonary emboli**, or **COPD** exacerbations. It is also common during **asthma** attacks, when the patient has difficulty breathing effectively due to bronchial obstruction. Polypnoea can also occur in response to **metabolic acidosis**, when the body attempts to eliminate excess acid in the form of carbon dioxide by increasing respiration, as seen in **unbalanced diabetes** (diabetic ketoacidosis).

Prolonged polypnoea can lead to **respiratory exhaustion**, as the respiratory muscles, particularly the diaphragm, eventually fatigue. If the underlying cause is not promptly treated, this can progress to **hypoventilation** and respiratory failure. Polypnoea is often accompanied by other clinical signs, such as tachycardia, excessive sweating and sometimes cyanosis, and requires rapid blood gas assessment to measure the extent of hypoxia or hypercapnia (accumulation of carbon dioxide).

  ◦ Measurements of vital constants: respiratory rate, O2 saturation

**Measuring vital constants** is an essential step in assessing a patient's state of health, particularly in pulmonology where respiratory function is often compromised. Among these constants, **respiratory rate** and **oxygen saturation** are two key indicators that monitor the patient's ability to breathe properly and oxygenate the blood. These measurements provide valuable information on lung function and the quality of gas exchange, and are often the first signs of respiratory decompensation or clinical improvement.

## Respiratory frequency

**Respiratory rate** is the number of breaths a patient takes per minute. In a healthy adult, this frequency is generally between **12 and 20 breaths per minute**. This vital constant is a direct indicator of respiratory effort and the body's response to possible distress or infection. Measuring respiratory rate is a simple but crucial act, often overlooked in care, when it can reveal important clinical information, long before other signs of respiratory distress become evident.

To measure respiratory rate, the caregiver or nurse counts the patient's breathing movements for a full minute, or for 30 seconds (multiplying by two). This procedure must be carried out in a calm environment, without the patient being aware of the observation, as he or she could involuntarily modify his or her breathing. A **high respiratory rate**, known as **polypnoea**, is often the first sign of respiratory distress. It occurs when the body tries to compensate for low oxygenation or excess carbon dioxide in the blood. This tachypnea can be observed during a lung infection (pneumonia), an exacerbation of COPD, or an asthma attack. A high respiratory rate indicates that the respiratory muscles are working harder to ensure adequate oxygenation.

Conversely, a **low respiratory rate**, known as **bradypnea**, may indicate respiratory depression, often associated with neurological damage, excessive use of sedative or opioid drugs, or extreme fatigue of the respiratory muscles after prolonged distress. This type of bradypnea is a cause for concern, as it means that gas exchange is not taking place properly, and the patient may go into **respiratory failure**.

In addition to simple frequency, the quality of breathing should also be observed. Shallow or irregular breathing may indicate increased respiratory effort or obstructive discomfort, as in asthma attacks or obstructive lung disease.

## Oxygen saturation (SpO2)

**Oxygen saturation** (SpO2) is another fundamental indicator of the lungs' ability to oxygenate the blood. It corresponds to the percentage of **hemoglobin** in the blood that is bound to oxygen. Oxygen saturation is measured using a **pulse oximeter**, a small device usually placed on the finger or earlobe. This device emits light beams through the skin and measures the absorption of light by oxygenated and deoxygenated hemoglobin, making it possible to calculate the percentage of oxygen saturation.

In a healthy individual, oxygen saturation is generally between **95% and 100%**. Lower values may indicate **hypoxemia**, i.e. insufficient oxygen in the blood. An SpO2 below **90%** is of particular concern, as it reflects a significant alteration in tissue and organ oxygenation. This drop can be caused by a variety of conditions, including pneumonia, COPD exacerbation, pulmonary edema, or acute pathologies such as pulmonary embolism or acute respiratory distress.

The pulse oximeter enables real-time monitoring of the patient's condition and early detection of hypoxemia, even before the appearance of visible clinical signs such as cyanosis. That's why this device is particularly useful in pneumology departments, but also in intensive care and emergency units.

When oxygen saturation is low, the first line of treatment is often **oxygen therapy**, which re-establishes adequate oxygen levels in the blood by administering oxygen via nasal cannula, mask, or in more severe cases, assisted ventilation. It is important to monitor saturation levels closely after oxygen therapy to ensure that oxygenation improves.

## The importance of regular monitoring

Measuring respiratory rate and oxygen saturation on a regular basis is essential to assess a patient's clinical evolution, whether in the acute phase of a respiratory pathology or in the recovery phase. These two constants must be assessed together, as they complement each other. For example, a patient in polypnoea with normal saturation may be in early respiratory distress, trying to compensate for incipient hypoxia. Conversely, a patient with a normal respiratory rate but low saturation needs immediate attention to understand and treat the cause of the hypoxia.

In addition, oxygen saturation monitoring is particularly useful in chronic respiratory diseases such as COPD or pulmonary fibrosis. In these patients, it is important to monitor changes in saturation, particularly during exercise, in order to adapt treatments such as home oxygen therapy or respiratory rehabilitation.

Finally, the caregiver must also be able to interpret the measurements in the overall context of the patient. For example, in some patients with severe COPD, saturations slightly below 90% may be tolerated if stable, as these patients often have chronically altered respiratory balance. However, any significant variation in respiratory rate or oxygen saturation should alert the health-care team and prompt a more thorough clinical reassessment.

- **Preparing the patient for pneumological examinations**
  ∘ Chest X-rays, CT scan, bronchial fibroscopy

Imaging and exploratory examinations such as **chest X-rays**, computed tomography (CT) scans and **bronchial fibroscopy** are essential tools in pulmonology for diagnosing, monitoring and evaluating various respiratory pathologies. These methods enable us to visualize the structures of the lungs, bronchial tubes and thoracic cavity, and provide valuable information on the condition of the airways and lung tissue. Each of these techniques has its own specificities and indications, and they are often complementary in the management of respiratory diseases.

## Chest X-ray

The **chest X-ray** is one of the most commonly used examinations in pulmonology to assess the condition of the lungs and rib cage structures. It is fast, inexpensive and non-invasive, and provides a comprehensive view of the lungs, heart, ribs and other thoracic structures. X-rays are generally taken from the front (posteroanterior view) and sometimes from the side, to obtain a more complete image of the lungs and mediastinum.

This examination is often the first diagnostic tool used when a patient presents respiratory symptoms such as cough, shortness of breath or chest pain. It can detect **visible abnormalities** such as **opacities** (areas of shadow in the lungs), **pleural effusions** (accumulation of fluid around the lungs), **pneumothorax** (presence of air in the pleural cavity), or suspicious **lesions** that may suggest lung cancer.

In the case of lung infections such as ,pneumonia the chest X-ray often shows pulmonary infiltrates, i.e. areas where the alveoli are filled with inflammatory fluid, resulting in an opacity on the image. In **COPD**, hyperinflation of the lungs, flattened diaphragms and widening of the mediastinum can be observed. In conditions such as **pulmonary fibrosis**, radiography can reveal diffuse changes, although this examination is often insufficient to fully assess the extent of the disease.

However, although radiography is a first-line tool, it has its limitations, particularly in detecting smaller or deeper lesions in the lungs. In these cases, more detailed examinations, such as a **chest CT scan**, are required to obtain a more accurate and complete picture.

## Chest CT scan (computed tomography)

The **thoracic CT scan**, or **computed tomography (CT)**, is an advanced imaging test that provides cross-sectional images of the thorax, enabling much finer and more detailed visualization than plain radiography. Using X-rays combined with computer techniques, CT creates three-dimensional images of the lungs, bronchi, mediastinum, blood vessels and adjacent structures.

CT scans are particularly useful for assessing abnormalities visible on X-ray, or for searching for lesions invisible on X-ray. In the case of **lung cancer**, for example, CT scans can be used to

73

detect nodules or smaller tumors, and to determine their location, size and relationship to surrounding structures. It is also used to search for **metastases** (spread of cancer to other parts of the body) or to guide lung biopsies.

In diseases such as **pulmonary fibrosis**, high-resolution CT (HR CT) is the gold standard, as it can visualize architectural changes in the lung with great precision, such as the **honeycomb** appearance (accumulation of cysts) characteristic of advanced fibrosis. This type of scan is also used to diagnose interstitial diseases, complex infections, or to assess the severity of pulmonary embolism, where it can show the presence of clots in the pulmonary arteries.

**Contrast-enhanced CT scanning** is sometimes used to better visualize blood vessels and assess pathologies such as pulmonary embolism or vascular malformations. Although this examination is more precise than radiography, it exposes the patient to a higher dose of X-rays and may require special precaution in patients with renal insufficiency due to the use of contrast medium.

## Bronchial fibroscopy

**Bronchial fibroscopy**, also known as **bronchoscopy**, is an endoscopic procedure that allows direct examination of the interior of the bronchi and airways, using a flexible tube equipped with a small camera. Unlike X-rays and CT scans, which provide images from the outside, bronchial fibroscopy enables direct visualization of the trachea, bronchi and large bronchioles, which is particularly useful for identifying abnormalities inside the airways.

This examination is indicated when suspicious lesions are visualized on an X-ray or CT scan, or when the patient presents symptoms such as **hemoptysis** (coughing up blood), **bronchial obstruction**, or signs of persistent infection despite treatment. Fibroscopy can identify **bronchial tumors**, **stenosis** (narrowing of the bronchi) or local **inflammation**. It is also useful for taking

**biopsies of** lung or bronchial tissue, to confirm the diagnosis of pathologies such as cancer, tuberculosis or specific lung infections.

In addition to its diagnostic role, bronchial fibroscopy can be used for **therapeutic** purposes. For example, it can be used to remove inhaled foreign bodies, aspirate mucus or fluid blocking the airways, or administer localized treatments such as bronchoalveolar lavage (instillation and aspiration of a fluid to clean the bronchial tubes and collect cells for analysis).

Bronchial fibroscopy is performed under local anesthesia (in the nose and throat) or general anesthesia, depending on the context and the patient's condition. Although the procedure is generally well tolerated, it may cause temporary discomfort, coughing fits or slight pain after the examination. In some cases, complications such as bleeding or infection may occur, although this is rare.

　　　◦　　Psychological and technical support
**Psychological and technical support** is an essential component of patient care, particularly in pneumology, where respiratory illnesses can have a profound impact on physical and emotional well-being. Whether chronic, such as COPD, or acute, such as pneumonia, these conditions can cause anxiety, distress and a sense of loss of control in patients. It is therefore essential that the care team not only focuses on the technical aspects of care, but also takes into account emotional support, creating a holistic, patient-centred care framework.

# Psychological support

**Psychological support** is based on a humanistic and empathetic approach, designed to help patients cope with their illness and mitigate its impact on their quality of life. Respiratory diseases can seriously affect patients' morale, especially when dyspnea (difficulty in breathing) becomes a distressing daily experience. Breathing is a vital function that we generally perform without thinking about it. But when it becomes difficult, it can generate immense stress, a fear of suffocation and, ultimately, lead to anxiety or depressive disorders.

The role of the healthcare team is therefore to provide ongoing **emotional support**, listening to patients' concerns and offering them a space in which to express their anxieties, doubts and frustrations. For example, a patient with advanced COPD may feel fearful about the future, fearing that he or she will become increasingly dependent on oxygen or lose autonomy. Appropriate psychological care involves listening to these fears, validating them, and offering clear answers about the course of the disease and management strategies. It is important to **acknowledge the** patient's **emotions** without minimizing his or her feelings, which strengthens the relationship of trust between caregiver and patient.

Psychological interventions may include sessions with **psychologists** or **psychiatrists**, particularly when the patient shows signs of severe anxiety or depression. **Relaxation** or **stress management** techniques, such as controlled breathing, can also be suggested to help the patient cope better with periods of acute dyspnoea. Indeed, the fear of running out of air can itself aggravate dyspnea, creating a vicious circle in which anxiety feeds breathing difficulties. Learning to use relaxation techniques, to control breathing or to practice mindfulness can help the patient to better manage these moments of crisis.

In the case of chronic respiratory illnesses, psychological care must also include support for the patient's loved ones. They often play an important role in day-to-day care, but may themselves be stressed or exhausted by their loved one's illness. Offering them advice, including them in discussions about care and providing them with resources to better understand the disease and how to help, is an integral part of overall psychological support.

# Technical support

**Technical support**, meanwhile, is essential to help patients understand and correctly use the various medical devices required to manage their respiratory pathology. These devices may include **oxygen therapy, non-invasive ventilation** (NIV), **inhalers** or **nebulizers**. While these devices are essential for the treatment of many respiratory diseases, they can also be a source of concern or discomfort for the patient, particularly if they are being used for the first time.

The role of the caregiver and the medical team is therefore to provide **clear, educational technical support**. This starts with a detailed explanation of why these devices are necessary. For example, explaining to a patient undergoing home oxygen therapy that the aim of this treatment is to compensate for the drop in oxygen in his blood will help him understand the importance of using the equipment correctly. Explanations must be simple, adapted to the patient's level of understanding, and accompanied by concrete demonstrations.

Secondly, technical support involves teaching the patient how to use the equipment correctly. This includes, for example, how to properly fit an oxygen mask or a non-invasive ventilation device, how to use a metered-dose inhaler, or how to maintain and clean these devices. In the case of **inhalers**, poor inhalation technique can considerably reduce the effectiveness of the treatment. The caregiver must therefore check that the patient has understood how to use the device, and if necessary correct the method by having the patient repeat the gestures.

Technical support also includes **monitoring** the patient's progress and the correct use of equipment over time. Adjustments may need to be made, for example, by increasing or decreasing the oxygen flow according to the patient's needs, or changing the device if the current one is no longer suitable. In some cases, the care team must ensure that the patient has the necessary material resources at home (such as portable oxygen tanks for travel) and knows when and how to use them.

This technical support aims to **empower** patients as much as possible. By mastering the use of their devices, patients become active players in their own care, which can considerably improve their quality of life and morale. This is particularly true for patients with chronic illnesses, who must learn to live with their treatment on a daily basis. Enabling them to manage their care at home, with greater confidence in the use of equipment, is a key objective of technical support.

# Chapter 4

# Daily care of the respiratory caregiver

- **Clinical monitoring of the patient**
  - ◦ Observation of signs of respiratory decompensation

**Observing the signs of respiratory decompensation** is a crucial step in the management of patients with acute or chronic respiratory diseases. Respiratory decompensation occurs when the body's own compensatory mechanisms, such as increased respiratory rate or use of accessory respiratory muscles, are no longer sufficient to maintain adequate oxygenation and efficient elimination of carbon dioxide. This situation leads to a progressive deterioration in gas exchange, with a significant risk of acute respiratory failure, sometimes fatal. Careful, systematic observation of the signs of decompensation enables rapid action to be taken, treatment to be adapted and serious complications to be avoided.

## Aggravated dyspnea

One of the first signs of respiratory decompensation is worsening **dyspnea** (shortness of breath), which becomes increasingly intense and persistent. The patient may report increasing difficulty in breathing, not only on exertion but also at rest, and experience chest tightness. Dyspnea, which was initially tolerated during certain activities, becomes incapacitating on a daily basis. Depending on the severity of the decompensation, the patient may adopt particular positions, such as **sitting leaning forward**, which helps maximize the function of the respiratory muscles, particularly the diaphragm. This sign should alert the care team, as it indicates that the patient's normal breathing is no longer sufficient to compensate for the body's oxygen requirements.

## Tachypnea and polypnea

Another important sign of respiratory decompensation is an **increase in respiratory rate**, known as **tachypnea** (abnormal increase in respiratory rate), or **polypnea** when respirations are rapid and shallow. The patient attempts to compensate for insufficient gas exchange by increasing the rate of breathing, but this strategy often only worsens the situation, as rapid, shallow breathing reduces the efficiency of gas exchange in the lungs. Persistent tachypnea is therefore a warning sign that must be taken seriously. The patient's oxygenation must be rapidly reassessed and adjusted if necessary.

## Use of accessory respiratory muscles

In the event of respiratory decompensation, the patient may be forced to use **accessory respiratory muscles** in an attempt to maintain adequate breathing. This can often be seen in exaggerated movements of the **intercostal, neck** and **shoulder muscles. Emphysema** and **COPD** are pathologies where this phenomenon is frequently observed. This is known as **draught**, a retraction of the intercostal spaces, supra-clavicular fossae or sternal fossa on inspiration. This sign indicates that the diaphragm, the main respiratory muscle, is no longer sufficient to ensure efficient breathing, and that the patient is exhausted trying to maintain correct oxygenation.

## Cyanosis

**Cyanosis** is one of the most serious physical signs of respiratory decompensation. It manifests as a **bluish** discoloration of the lips, nails or face, and reflects a lack of oxygen in the blood (**hypoxemia**). This sign indicates a significant deterioration in gas exchange and generalized hypoxia, i.e. the body's tissues no longer receive enough oxygen to function properly. Cyanosis is an indicator of a medical emergency, requiring immediate attention. Oxygen therapy or assisted ventilation is often required to restore adequate oxygenation levels.

## Altered state of consciousness

Respiratory failure can also lead to **altered consciousness**. When the brain lacks oxygen (cerebral hypoxia) or the level of carbon dioxide in the blood (hypercapnia) increases, the patient may become **confused**, **agitated** or even **drowsy**. In more advanced stages, this can progress to unconsciousness. This sign is often underestimated, but it indicates impending respiratory failure. Psychomotor agitation or excessive somnolence should therefore be closely monitored, requiring immediate reassessment of the patient's blood gases and respiratory status.

## Hypoxemia and oxygen saturation

**Oxygen saturation** (SpO2) is a fundamental indicator of patient oxygenation. Normal saturation is between 95% and 100%. When saturation falls below 90%, this is **hypoxemia**, which may signal respiratory decompensation. Hypoxemia leads to poor oxygenation of vital organs, and if it persists, can cause multiple organ failure. Regular measurement of oxygen saturation, using a pulse oximeter, is therefore essential to monitor the patient's progress. Any sudden drop in saturation requires immediate intervention, often with oxygen therapy or mechanical ventilation if conventional oxygen therapy is not sufficient.

## Blood gas anomalies

**Blood gases** are a key test for assessing a patient's respiratory status and gas exchange capacity. In the event of respiratory decompensation, a blood gas analysis often shows **hypoxemia** (decrease in the partial pressure of oxygen in arterial blood), sometimes associated with **hypercapnia** (increase in the partial pressure of carbon dioxide). Hypercapnia is particularly common in diseases such as COPD, where carbon dioxide elimination is compromised. In addition to these abnormalities, **respiratory acidosis** can occur when the inability to eliminate $CO_2$ leads to acidification of the blood, making the situation even worse. Blood gas monitoring can assess the severity of decompensation and guide the initiation of non-invasive ventilation or other more invasive interventions.

◦ Respiratory parameters to monitor (saturation, breath sounds)

**Monitoring respiratory parameters** is essential for assessing a patient's state of health, particularly in pulmonology. Among these parameters, **oxygen saturation (SpO2)** and **breath sounds** are two key elements for assessing respiratory function and detecting early signs of respiratory distress. These indicators provide both objective information (such as saturation values) and subjective information (through auscultation of breath sounds), and their rigorous monitoring enables treatments to be adjusted early and effectively.

## Oxygen saturation (SpO2)

**Oxygen saturation**, or SpO2, measures the percentage of hemoglobin in the blood that is saturated with oxygen. It is a direct indicator of the capacity of the lungs to oxygenate the blood, and of the gas exchanges taking place in the pulmonary alveoli. Normally, in a healthy person, saturation is between **95% and 100%**. Saturation below these values indicates **hypoxemia**, i.e. a lack of oxygen in the blood, often requiring immediate intervention.

Oxygen saturation is measured non-invasively using a **pulse oximeter**, a device usually placed on the fingertip, earlobe or, in some cases, on the nose. This device works by emitting beams of light through the skin, measuring the amount of oxygen bound to hemoglobin. This measurement is invaluable for monitoring acute or chronic respiratory diseases, such as **pneumonia, COPD, asthma or pulmonary fibrosis**, where the lungs' ability to oxygenate the blood may be compromised.

An oxygen saturation of less than **90%** is particularly worrying, and signals **potential respiratory failure**. In such cases, the body is no longer able to ensure proper oxygenation, which can lead to symptoms such as **dyspnea** (shortness of breath), **cyanosis** (bluish discoloration of the skin and mucous membranes) and **tachycardia**. Low saturation may require the administration of supplementary oxygen via oxygen therapy or, in more serious situations, **assisted ventilation**.

In addition to absolute saturation values, it is essential to monitor **variations** over time. A rapid fall in SpO2, especially if associated with an increase in respiratory rate or visible respiratory discomfort, should alert the nursing team. In patients with chronic respiratory diseases, such as COPD, it may be necessary to adapt expectations. In these patients, saturation levels slightly below 90% can be tolerated, but any deterioration must be carefully monitored.

**Nocturnal saturation** is also a parameter to consider, particularly in patients suffering from conditions such as sleep apnea, COPD or heart failure. Nocturnal desaturation, i.e. a fall in SpO2 during sleep, may indicate a nocturnal ventilation problem and often requires further evaluation, including tests such as **polysomnography**.

## Breathing sounds

**Respiratory sounds** are another fundamental parameter to monitor. **Pulmonary auscultation**, performed with a stethoscope, makes it possible to hear the sounds produced by the air circulating in the lungs and bronchi. Auscultation enables us to assess the quality of breathing, detect abnormalities and guide the diagnosis of lung pathologies.

In a healthy person, breath sounds are **clear** and **symmetrical** on both sides of the chest. However, in the presence of respiratory pathologies, various **abnormal noises** can be heard, indicating airway obstruction, inflammation, or the presence of fluid in the alveoli.

- **Crackles**: These fine noises, often described as crinkling paper or bursting bubbles, are usually heard during inspiration. They are associated with the presence of fluid or mucus in the alveoli, and may indicate conditions such as **pneumonia**, **pulmonary edema** or **pulmonary fibrosis**. Crackles can be **dry** or **wet**, depending on the underlying cause.

- **Sibilance**: Sibilance is a high-pitched whistling sound, heard mainly during exhalation. They indicate partial bronchial obstruction, often due to **bronchoconstriction** in conditions such as **asthma** or **COPD**. Their intensity and location can vary according to the severity of airway constriction.

- **Ronchi**: Ronchi are low, gurgling-like noises heard during exhalation. They are caused by the accumulation of secretions in the large bronchi. They are often associated with lower respiratory tract infections, such as **bronchitis** or viral infections, and may disappear after a productive cough.

- **Stridor**: Stridor is a high-pitched respiratory noise heard mainly during inspiration, and is often a sign of upper airway obstruction, as in the case of a foreign body or severe laryngeal edema. This sound is a medical emergency, requiring rapid intervention to clear the airways.

In addition to these abnormal sounds, the absence or reduction of respiratory sounds in any part of the chest can also be a warning sign. This may indicate the presence of a **pneumothorax** (air in the pleural cavity), **pleural effusion** (accumulation of fluid around the lungs), or severe bronchial obstruction.

## Importance of regular monitoring

**Oxygen saturation** and **breath sounds** can be monitored to assess the evolution of respiratory pathologies and to adjust treatments according to the patient's needs. In the presence of low saturation or abnormal breath sounds, rapid intervention can prevent serious complications such as acute respiratory decompensation. Regular, even continuous monitoring is essential for some patients, to anticipate oxygen requirements, therapeutic adjustments, or the need for additional tests such as chest X-rays or scans.

○ Monitoring patients on oxygen therapy

**Monitoring patients on oxygen therapy** is an essential part of the management of chronic or acute respiratory illnesses. Oxygen therapy, whether short- or long-term, compensates for respiratory insufficiency by delivering extra oxygen to the lungs and, consequently, to the blood. However, this treatment, though effective, requires regular and rigorous monitoring to ensure that it is correctly adapted to the patient's needs, well tolerated, and genuinely improves quality of life and respiratory health. Monitoring focuses on both clinical and technical aspects, to ensure optimal use of oxygen while minimizing risks and complications.

## Oxygen saturation monitoring

One of the key aspects of monitoring patients on oxygen therapy is regular monitoring of **oxygen saturation (SpO2)**, which directly reflects the effectiveness of the treatment. Oxygen saturation is measured using a pulse oximeter, a non-invasive device that provides a percentage reading of blood oxygenation levels. In patients on oxygen therapy, the aim is generally to maintain an SpO2 between **88%** **and 92%** in patients with chronic diseases such as COPD, or between **95%** **and 98%** in patients with acute respiratory failure. It is crucial to adapt oxygen flow to the measured saturation to avoid both hypoxia (oxygen deficiency) and hyperoxia (oxygen excess), the latter of which can lead to complications, particularly in COPD patients.

SpO2 monitoring must be particularly careful when initiating oxygen therapy, after any flow adjustment, and when the patient presents unusual symptoms, such as worsening dyspnea, headaches or signs of cyanosis. Continuous monitoring, with frequent readings, ensures that oxygen is being administered adequately and that the patient's needs are being met, both at rest and during exercise.

## Regular clinical assessment

Clinical assessment of the patient on oxygen therapy is also essential to ensure that the treatment is actually improving the patient's respiratory condition. The care team, in collaboration with the pulmonary physician, must closely monitor **clinical signs** such as **dyspnea**, **respiratory rate**, **fatigue** and **sleep quality**. Dyspnea is often one of the first symptoms improved by oxygen therapy, and patients should be asked about changes in their ability to perform physical activities, such as walking or climbing stairs.

In addition to assessing breathing, it's important to watch for symptoms that could indicate complications from oxygen therapy, such as chest pain, headache or sleep disturbance, especially in patients with hypercapnia (accumulation of $CO_2$ in the blood). Regular **blood gas** examinations may be necessary to assess the presence of hypercapnia or respiratory acidosis, especially in patients at risk of $CO_2$ retention, such as those with severe COPD. This monitoring enables oxygen flow rates to be adjusted or a switch made to more advanced devices, such as non-invasive ventilation (NIV), if oxygen therapy alone is not sufficient to maintain adequate oxygenation levels without risk of $CO_2$ retention.

## Oxygen flow adaptation

One of the main aims of monitoring is to adjust the **oxygen flow** to the patient's needs. The oxygen flow rate initially prescribed by the doctor may need to be modified over time, depending on the patient's clinical progress and the results of oxygen saturation monitoring. The caregiver or nurse must regularly check that the oxygen flow rate is correctly set on the equipment and corresponds to the medical prescription. For some patients, the need for oxygen may vary according to activity: a higher flow rate may be required during physical exertion, such as walking, while a lower flow rate may be sufficient at rest.

For patients on long-term oxygen therapy, **regular reassessment** of the need for oxygen therapy and the flow rates required is essential. Such reassessments are recommended every three to six months, or more frequently if the patient's condition changes. In some cases, therapy can be adjusted or even reduced if the patient's condition improves.

## Monitoring compliance and use of equipment

Therapeutic **compliance** is a crucial aspect of monitoring patients on home oxygen therapy. Some patients may find it difficult to use their equipment correctly, either because of discomfort (prolonged wearing of nasal cannula or mask), unfamiliarity with instructions, or discomfort linked to oxygen dependency. The care team must regularly check that the patient understands how to use the equipment, knows how to adjust the oxygen flow and is using the devices correctly (nasal cannula, face masks, oxygen concentrators). Technical support is therefore essential to ensure that patients are comfortable with their equipment, and that they clean and maintain it correctly.

In addition, it's important to discuss the patient's **day-to-day experience** with oxygen therapy on a regular basis, addressing any difficulties or side-effects experienced. This enables the treatment to be adapted to the patient's feedback. Regular exchanges can also help reinforce compliance by explaining the long-term benefits of oxygen therapy and dispelling any doubts or misgivings the patient may have.

# Monitoring potential complications

Oxygen therapy, while life-saving for many patients, is not without its risks. **Drying of the** nasal **mucosa** is a frequent side effect, especially if oxygen is administered at a high flow rate without humidification. The care-health team should monitor for the appearance of irritation or lesions in the nostrils, and provide advice on how to alleviate this discomfort, for example by recommending oxygen humidification solutions or suitable nasal care. Other potential complications include infections linked to improper use or inadequate maintenance of the devices, hence the importance of rigorous training and technical follow-up.

Finally, **hyperoxia** can be a serious complication, especially in patients with COPD or pathologies associated with $CO_2$ retention. Excessive oxygen administration in these patients can lead to deterioration in their respiratory function by reducing their natural respiratory stimulus, thereby aggravating hypercapnia. For this reason, blood gas monitoring and SpO2 monitoring are essential to avoid these complications.

- **Managing dyspnea and respiratory fatigue**
  - Postures to improve ventilation

**Postures to improve ventilation** are specific positions that patients can adopt to facilitate breathing, optimizing the function of the lungs and respiratory muscles. These positions are particularly useful for patients suffering from chronic respiratory diseases, such as **COPD, asthma** or **heart failure**, or during acute attacks of respiratory distress, such as exacerbations of COPD or pneumonia. These postures reduce respiratory effort, improve gas exchange in the lungs and relieve symptoms of breathlessness.

## Sitting leaning forward

One of the most effective postures for improving ventilation is the **forward-leaning sitting position**, also known as the **tripod position**. In this position, the patient sits with a slight forward tilt, elbows resting on knees or a low table, hands on thighs or a stable surface. This posture is commonly adopted by **COPD** patients during dyspnea attacks.

This position relieves pressure on the main **respiratory muscles**, in particular the **diaphragm**, allowing it to move more freely and efficiently during inspiration. Sitting and leaning, intra-abdominal pressure is reduced, giving the diaphragm more room to contract and relax. In addition, this posture allows the accessory muscles of respiration, such as the intercostal and neck muscles, to be more active, helping to compensate for the respiratory effort required to inhale more air.

This posture is often instinctively adopted by patients in respiratory distress, as it rapidly relieves the sensation of breathlessness by reducing the load on the lungs and facilitating airflow. It can be particularly useful during acute exacerbations of obstructive lung disease, such as **COPD** or **asthma**, or in **heart failure** patients with pulmonary congestion.

## The semi-seated position (Fowler)

The **semi-seated** or **Fowler position** is another classic posture for improving ventilation, particularly in bedridden patients. In this position, the patient lies with the torso inclined at an angle of **45 to 60 degrees** to the horizontal, legs slightly elevated to promote good blood circulation. This posture optimizes breathing while remaining in a resting position.

The Fowler position is often used in hospital settings for patients with breathing difficulties, as it reduces the pressure exerted by the abdominal organs on the diaphragm, facilitating its movement and increasing lung capacity. It is particularly beneficial for patients suffering from **pneumonia, pulmonary fibrosis** or recovering from thoracic surgery. By reducing breathlessness, this position improves the patient's ability to ventilate the lungs more efficiently, and helps prevent **atelectasis** (collapse of the alveoli).

This posture is also useful in **congestive heart failure**, where patients often suffer from **orthopnea**, a form of dyspnea that occurs in the supine position. By keeping the patient in a semi-seated position, pressure on the lungs is reduced, facilitating pulmonary expansion and reducing the sensation of chest tightness.

## Prone position

The **prone position**, or **proning**, involves the patient lying on his or her stomach, arms by his or her sides or slightly elevated, with the head tilted to one side. This posture is increasingly used in cases of severe respiratory distress, particularly in intensive care units, for patients suffering from **acute respiratory distress syndrome (ARDS)** or **severe respiratory failure**.

The main advantage of this position is that it improves **air distribution** throughout the lungs, particularly in the posterior zones, which are often less well ventilated when lying on the back. In the prone position, the weight of the heart and abdominal organs exerts less pressure on the lungs, enabling better **alveolar expansion** and more efficient gas exchange. This position also promotes drainage of secretions, helping to reduce the risk of pulmonary complications such as **infection** or **atelectasis**.

**Proning** is particularly effective for improving oxygenation in mechanically ventilated patients in intensive care, but can also be beneficial for non-intubated patients suffering from moderate hypoxemia. However, this position must be used with caution and under supervision, particularly in patients with hemodynamic disorders or pressure-sensitive wounds.

## Lying on your side (lateral decubitus)

The **lateral decubitus position**, where the patient lies on his or her side, can also be useful for improving ventilation, especially in patients with unilateral lung involvement, such as in cases of **pneumonia** or **atelectasis involving** a single lung. In this position, it is advisable to lie the patient on the **unaffected** side. This posture enables the healthy lung to receive greater blood flow, optimizing gas exchange.

Lateral decubitus is often recommended to improve patient comfort, facilitate postural drainage of secretions and reduce breathlessness in bedridden patients. This position is also beneficial in the management of chronic respiratory diseases, such as COPD, where patients may need to change position regularly to avoid secretion stasis and maintain adequate ventilation.

## Mobilization and breathing exercises

In addition to specific postures, it's important to encourage patients to **mobilize regularly** and practice **breathing exercises**. Simple movements, such as standing up and walking even short distances, can improve ventilation by stimulating the diaphragm and promoting better aeration of the lungs. **Diaphragmatic** or **pursed-lip breathing** exercises are often taught to patients to improve breathing efficiency and reduce dyspnoea.

These techniques strengthen respiratory muscles, optimize alveolar ventilation and promote secretion elimination, thereby reducing the risk of respiratory infections and complications. For patients who are bedridden or less mobile, **respiratory physiotherapy** exercises can be performed to maintain good lung function.

○ Support in managing daily effort

**Support in managing daily effort** is essential for patients with chronic respiratory diseases, such as **COPD, severe asthma, pulmonary fibrosis**, or those in remission after acute pathologies such as pneumonia. These patients are faced with physical limitations that impact on their ability to carry out activities of daily living, such as walking, washing, climbing stairs or simply talking without being out of breath. To maintain optimal quality of life and prevent exacerbations, it is crucial to support them in learning strategies and techniques to effectively manage their daily physical effort.

## The importance of personalized assessment

Before proposing a support plan, it is essential to carry out a **personalized assessment of** the patient's physical capacity, taking into account the severity of his respiratory pathology, his level of exercise tolerance and his specific needs. This assessment enables us to better understand the patient's limitations and adapt our interventions accordingly. For example, a patient with **moderate COPD** may be encouraged to walk short distances with frequent breaks, while a patient with **advanced pulmonary fibrosis** may need mobile oxygen therapy to carry out simple activities without becoming exhausted.

This assessment also takes into account the **emotional repercussions** of these physical limitations. Fear of breathlessness, effort-related anxiety, and sometimes even depression, can lead patients to limit their physical activity. Effort management support therefore includes psychological support to help them overcome these fears and restore their confidence in their ability to be active.

## Breathing management techniques

One of the first steps in helping patients to better manage daily effort is to teach them appropriate **breathing techniques**. These techniques optimize breathing and reduce the sensation of breathlessness, particularly during physical activity.

- **Pursed-lip breathing**: This technique involves breathing slowly in through the nose and gently out through the mouth, pursing the lips slightly as if blowing through a straw. This method helps to **prolong exhalation**, enabling carbon dioxide to be removed from the lungs more efficiently, which is particularly beneficial for patients suffering from bronchial obstruction such as COPD. It also reduces breathlessness during exercise, making physical activity more tolerable.

- **Diaphragmatic breathing**: Also known as abdominal breathing, this technique relies on the use of the diaphragm, the main breathing muscle, rather than the accessory muscles of the upper chest. The patient is encouraged to inhale deeply by inflating the abdomen, then exhale slowly by relaxing it. This improves **alveolar ventilation** and reduces breathlessness during exercise. This technique can be particularly useful before and during strenuous activities such as climbing stairs or carrying objects.

## Business planning and management

One of the keys to helping patients better manage their daily effort is to encourage them to **plan their activities so as** to spread effort throughout the day. This includes prioritizing the most important tasks and interspersing rest periods between each activity. The idea is to avoid burning out by carrying out several consecutive tasks without a break.

For example, for a patient who has difficulty standing for long periods, it is advisable to group together tasks that can be carried out in a seated position, such as brushing teeth or peeling vegetables. Similarly, it is useful to encourage the patient to avoid over-demanding activities immediately after meals, as digestion increases oxygen requirements and can aggravate the feeling of fatigue.

**Travel** management is also a priority. It is advisable to keep journeys short, or to break up long distances by stopping regularly to catch your breath. The use of **technical aids** such as a cane, walker or shopping cart can also be suggested, to take the strain off the body while enabling the patient to remain active.

## Encouraging appropriate physical activity

It may seem counter-intuitive to recommend exercise to patients suffering from breathlessness, but **adapted physical activity** is actually beneficial for improving exercise tolerance and quality of life. Regular exercise helps **strengthen the respiratory** and peripheral **muscles**, which in turn reduces the breathlessness experienced during physical activity. Moderate physical activity also improves blood circulation, enabling oxygen to be transported more efficiently throughout the body.

Exercises should be adapted to the patient's abilities and introduced gradually. **Gentle** activities such as walking, swimming or exercise cycling may be recommended, under the supervision of a physiotherapist or specialized coach. It is essential to start with short sessions lasting 5 to 10 minutes, then gradually increase the duration according to the patient's tolerance. **Breathing exercises** can be combined to optimize the use of lung capacity during exercise.

Participation in **respiratory rehabilitation programs** is also highly recommended. These supervised programs offer personalized support and enable patients to learn how to manage exertion while surrounded by professionals. They include physical exercise sessions, breathing techniques and advice on managing effort and symptoms on a daily basis.

## Use of oxygen therapy devices

For patients suffering from **hypoxemia** or **advanced COPD**, the use of **oxygen therapy** may be essential to maintain good oxygenation during physical exertion. It is important to ensure that patients know how to use their oxygen correctly, especially during exercise. The care team must ensure that patients understand how to adjust their oxygen flow during more demanding tasks, such as climbing stairs or walking long distances. In addition, the use of a **portable oxygen concentrator** enables patients to remain mobile and pursue outdoor activities without fear of blood oxygen desaturation.

## Psychological support

Managing daily effort can lead to **frustration** and **anxiety**, especially for patients who feel limited by their illness. It is therefore important to provide psychological support to help them overcome these feelings. Support should aim to restore their **self-confidence** and show them that they can continue to be active despite their respiratory difficulties. Support groups or sessions with a psychologist can help cope with anxiety linked to breathlessness and fear of exhaustion.

- **Hygiene care for respiratory patients**
  - Grooming and pressure sore prevention in bedridden patients

**Grooming** and **pressure sore prevention** for bedridden patients are essential in the hospital or at home, particularly for patients with reduced mobility. The aim is not only to maintain optimal personal hygiene, but also to prevent complications associated with prolonged immobility, such as **pressure sores**. Pressure sores develop when the skin and underlying tissues are subjected to continuous pressure, leading to poor blood circulation and tissue necrosis. Caregivers therefore have a dual objective: to ensure patient comfort, while adopting preventive measures to protect the skin and promote general well-being.

## Toileting the bedridden patient: fundamental care

**Toileting the bedridden patient** is a key moment, not only for maintaining cleanliness, but also for preserving the integrity of the skin, stimulating blood circulation and offering the patient a moment of comfort and well-being. It's a delicate task that requires attention, gentleness and constant communication with the patient to respect his or her dignity and privacy.

The caregiver begins by **preparing** the **equipment**: washcloth, mild soap or grease-free cleansing gel, towels, a basin of warm water, and, if necessary, moisturizing creams or suitable skin care products. The use of mild soap is crucial, as overly aggressive or drying soaps can irritate the fragile skin of bedridden patients, which is often more sensitive due to prolonged immobility or medical treatments. Moisturizing products are also recommended after cleansing to maintain skin suppleness and prevent dryness.

Washing is carried out **zone by zone**, ensuring that the patient is covered as much as possible to avoid the sensation of cold and to preserve privacy. The caregiver generally starts with the face and works progressively towards other parts of the body. Skin folds, such as the armpits, groin and under women's breasts, need to be cleansed with care, as they are areas prone to maceration, which promotes skin infections.

One of the important purposes of grooming is to enable the caregiver to **inspect the condition of** the patient's **skin**. Any redness, irritation or suspicious areas should be reported immediately, as they may be an early sign of pressure sore formation. Particular attention should be paid to bony areas of the body, such as the heels, sacrum, hips, elbows and shoulder blades,

97

as these are the areas most at risk of pressure sores due to the pressure exerted during immobilization.

## Pressure sore prevention: a priority issue

The **prevention of pressure sores** is an essential component of care for bedridden patients. Pressure sores form as a result of continuous pressure exerted on certain parts of the body, preventing proper blood circulation and causing tissue degradation. They most often appear on **bony areas**, where the skin is thinner and the weight of the body exerts significant pressure, such as the heels, sacrum, hips or elbows.

### Regular mobilization

One of the main ways of preventing pressure sores is to **mobilize** the patient on **a regular basis**. By frequently changing the patient's position, we reduce the constant pressure on certain areas and promote better blood circulation. We recommend **changing the patient's position every two hours**, depending on tolerance and comfort. This may include moving from lying on the back to lateral decubitus positions (on the side), alternating sides.

If the patient is able to participate in his or her own mobilization, he or she is encouraged to make small, regular movements, such as bending the legs or lifting the pelvis slightly, thus reducing pressure on certain areas. The use of a **bed lifter** can also enable the patient to use his or her arms to partially lift the body and change position.

### Use of prevention equipment

The use of **anti-bedsore mattresses and cushions** is another essential element in the prevention of pressure ulcers. These devices are specially designed to distribute pressure evenly over the whole body, preventing it from concentrating on vulnerable areas. Dynamic air mattresses, which alternate pressure points, are often used for high-risk patients. Cushions or heel pads can also be placed under heels or other high-risk areas to relieve pressure.

**Positioning cushions** are also useful to help keep the patient in a comfortable position and avoid friction and shearing, which can also contribute to pressure sore formation. These accessories are placed under the legs, between the knees or at arm level to ensure ergonomic support.

## Moisturizing and skin care

**Skin hydration** plays a vital role in preventing pressure sores. Well-moisturized skin is more supple and resistant to pressure. After cleansing, we recommend applying **moisturizing creams** or oils, particularly to at-risk areas, to preserve skin elasticity. Moisturizers should be light and non-occlusive, to allow the skin to breathe and avoid maceration.

It's also crucial to **prevent excessive humidity**, which can promote maceration and infections. Incontinent patients, for example, are particularly at risk, as moisture from urine or feces can quickly irritate the skin. So it's important to change absorbent pads regularly, maintain frequent cleansing and use barrier creams that protect the skin from irritation caused by moisture.

## Monitoring early signs

**Careful**, daily **monitoring** of the patient's skin enables early detection of early signs of pressure sore formation. Early signs include persistent **redness** that doesn't go away after decompressing the area, areas of hardened skin, or a change in skin texture or color. At this stage, prompt intervention can prevent progression to ulceration.

If signs of ulceration are observed, such as blisters, open wounds or necrotic areas, it is imperative to inform the medical team immediately so that appropriate treatment can be put in place, which may include specific dressings and wound care.

**Preventing nosocomial infections in the respiratory environment** is a major challenge in healthcare establishments, particularly in pneumology and intensive care units. These infections, contracted during the hospital stay, are often linked to the use of respiratory medical devices or exposure to infectious agents present in the hospital environment. They can lead to serious complications, particularly in vulnerable patients suffering from chronic respiratory pathologies or acute respiratory failure. Preventing these infections requires a rigorous approach, based on strict hygiene protocols, appropriate management of medical devices and increased surveillance.

## Hand hygiene: the first line of defense

**Hand hygiene** is one of the simplest and most effective measures for preventing nosocomial infections, and is particularly crucial in respiratory environments. Caregivers, as well as visitors and patients themselves, must wash their hands regularly to prevent the spread of germs. Nosocomial respiratory infections, such as **ventilator-associated pneumonia (VAP)**, can be caused by bacteria transmitted via contaminated hands.

Hands must be washed before and after every contact with the patient, before handling respiratory medical devices (such as oxygen masks, tubing or respirators), and after any procedure involving the risk of contamination. The use of hydroalcoholic solutions is recommended as a matter of routine, except when hands are visibly soiled, when washing with soap and water is essential. Although apparently simple, this practice must be strictly applied, as it plays a crucial role in reducing the transmission of pathogens in the hospital environment.

## Sterilization and disinfection of medical devices

**Rigorous sterilization and disinfection of medical devices** used in the respiratory environment are essential to prevent nosocomial

100

infections. Respiratory devices, such as ventilators, masks, intubation cannulas or nebulizers, can be important vectors for the transmission of bacteria and viruses if they are not properly disinfected.

Reusable equipment, such as tubing, oxygen masks or mechanical ventilator parts, must be cleaned, disinfected or sterilized according to strict protocols after each use, to eliminate all traces of microbial contaminants. Single-use devices, such as certain filters and tubing, must be properly disposed of after use to avoid cross-contamination between patients.

The use of **antimicrobial filters** in mechanical ventilators is another important measure for limiting the transmission of infectious agents. These filters, placed between the patient circuit and the device, retain potentially pathogenic particles, thus reducing the risk of cross-contamination.

## Management of ventilators and oxygen therapy devices

Patients undergoing **mechanical ventilation** or **prolonged oxygen therapy** are particularly at risk of contracting nosocomial infections, due to the invasion of devices into their airways. **Ventilator-associated pneumonia (VAP)** is one of the most frequent and serious nosocomial infections in intensive care, as the airways are directly exposed to external pathogens.

To reduce this risk, a number of preventive measures are required. First and foremost, we recommend keeping the patient in a **semi-seated** position, with the chest slightly inclined (30 to 45 degrees). This position reduces the risk of **inhalation of gastric secretions** into the lungs, a major factor in the development of nosocomial pneumonia.

Secondly, it is essential to **manage** the patient's **secretions**. Regular suctioning of bronchial secretions must be carried out using sterile equipment, to clear the airways without introducing germs. **Humidification of inspired air**, often necessary in patients on ventilation or oxygen therapy, must be controlled and monitored to avoid drying out the mucous membranes, while taking care not to encourage bacterial proliferation through excess humidity.

## Antibiotic prophylaxis and antibiotic stewardship

The rational use of **antibiotics** is another key element in the prevention of nosocomial infections in the respiratory environment. Inappropriate or excessive antibiotic therapy can encourage the emergence of **resistant bacteria**, responsible for nosocomial infections that are difficult to treat, such as **methicillin-resistant Staphylococcus aureus (MRSA)** or **resistant Enterobacteriaceae**.

Antibiotic prophylaxis, i.e. the preventive administration of antibiotics to high-risk patients (such as those undergoing mechanical ventilation), must be used sparingly and according to strict protocols. Antibiotics must be selected according to the **germs most frequently encountered** in the hospital environment, and administered for a limited duration to reduce the risk of resistance.

Regular **microbiological monitoring** of patients undergoing mechanical ventilation or oxygen therapy is essential for early detection of signs of infection and adaptation of treatment. Respiratory samples )bronchial aspirates or bronchoalveolar lavage) are used to identify pathogens and target antibiotic therapy.

## Hospital environment hygiene

The hospital environment itself can be a source of **cross-contamination**. Pathogens can survive on surfaces for prolonged periods and be transmitted from one patient to another by nursing staff, medical equipment or even everyday objects. Particular attention must be paid to **surface hygiene**, especially in intensive care or pneumology areas where high-risk patients are hospitalized.

**Frequently touched surfaces**, such as door handles, bed rails, tables and medical equipment, must be disinfected regularly using disinfectant products effective against bacteria, viruses and fungi. Cleaning protocols must be rigorously followed, with products adapted to each surface and cleaning frequencies adapted to the activity of the departments.

Caregivers must also be trained in the importance of **environmental hygiene**, particularly when handling respiratory medical devices. For example, caregivers must ensure that ventilator air filters are replaced regularly, and that oxygen therapy equipment is properly stored and maintained.

## Vaccination and patient isolation

Finally, **vaccination of** patients and nursing staff is an important preventive measure. Hospitalized patients, especially those with chronic respiratory pathologies, need to be **vaccinated against influenza** and **pneumococcus**, two agents responsible for many nosocomial respiratory infections. Nursing staff must also be vaccinated to limit the risk of transmitting viral infections such as influenza.

If a patient with a nosocomial infection, such as resistant pneumonia, is detected, it is crucial to implement **isolation** measures to prevent the spread of infection to other patients. This includes the use of personal protective equipment (gloves, gowns, masks), confinement of the patient to an individual room, and strict limitation of visits.

- **Nutrition and hydration aid**
  - Adapting diet to dyspnea

**Adapting diet to dyspnoea** is an essential component in the management of patients suffering from chronic respiratory diseases such as **COPD, severe asthma, pulmonary fibrosis** or **heart failure**. Dyspnoea, which translates into difficulty in breathing, can make mealtimes stressful for patients, to the point of leading to reduced appetite, malnutrition and even muscle wasting, which further aggravates respiratory failure. Adapting diet to these respiratory difficulties is therefore crucial to maintaining good nutritional status and avoiding a vicious circle in which dyspnea, fatigue and malnutrition reinforce each other.

## The impact of dyspnea on diet

**Dyspnea** directly affects the ability to eat comfortably and efficiently. Breathless patients may find it difficult to breathe and eat at the same time, as breathing and swallowing involve the same anatomical pathways. This may lead them to avoid meals or reduce their portions for fear of running out of air while eating. What's more, the extra effort required to breathe can exhaust patients, diminishing their appetite and motivation to eat, which can lead to involuntary **weight loss, muscle weakness** and a deterioration in general condition.

Another effect of dyspnea on eating is that some patients may be prone to **bloating** or **gastric discomfort**. The rapid ingestion of food, particularly when associated with difficult breathing, can lead to excessive swallowing of air (aerophagia), exacerbating the sensation of discomfort and chest tightness.

## Adapt meals to respiratory capacity

To help dyspneic patients maintain an adequate diet, a number of adjustments can be made to meal preparation, composition and frequency. These adaptations help reduce the physical and respiratory effort required during meals, while ensuring adequate nutritional intake.

## Split meals

One of the first pieces of advice for patients suffering from dyspnea is to **break up meals into** smaller portions spread throughout the day. Rather than eating three large meals, which can be exhausting and tiring, it is preferable to offer **five to six small**, light and frequent **meals**. This allows the patient to eat without feeling out of breath, and avoids the sensation of overloading the stomach, which can compress the diaphragm and aggravate dyspnea. In addition, this method helps avoid digestion-related fatigue, which can be particularly marked in respiratory patients.

## Choose foods that are easy to chew and swallow

Food should be **easy to chew and swallow,** to reduce the effort required during meals. Dyspneic patients may experience significant fatigue during chewing, prompting them to abandon their meal quickly. It is therefore advisable to prefer **soft** or **chopped** textures, such as vegetable purées, fruit compotes, soups or tender stews. These preparations require less muscular effort and allow you to eat without overtaxing your respiratory muscles.

Dry or hard-to-chew foods, such as crusty bread, hard meats or fibrous foods, should be avoided or eaten in small quantities. Protein- and calorie-rich **milkshakes** and **smoothies** can be interesting alternatives, as they provide the necessary nutrients while being easier to swallow.

## Avoid heavy, high-fat meals

**Overeating** or **high-fat** meals can lead to slow, heavy digestion, increasing the body's energy and respiratory demands. In addition, fatty meals can lead to bloating and abdominal discomfort, compressing the diaphragm and aggravating the sensation of breathlessness. It is therefore advisable to choose **light, easy-to-digest** foods, with a moderate amount of fat, while taking care to maintain a sufficient caloric intake to avoid weight loss. Fiber-rich meals, while beneficial for digestion, should be introduced with care to avoid bloating.

It's also best to **reduce consumption of carbonated beverages** and foods that promote aerophagia, as excessive ingestion of air can increase abdominal pressure and lead to further respiratory discomfort.

### Ensuring adequate calorie intake

**Malnutrition** is a major risk in dyspneic patients, as the combination of labored breathing and reduced appetite often leads to involuntary weight loss. This loss of weight, and in particular muscle mass, can worsen respiratory function, as respiratory muscles become weaker. It is therefore essential to **maintain an adequate caloric intake**, even when the patient finds it difficult to eat large quantities.

Meals should be **calorie-dense** and **nutrient-dense** to provide sufficient nutrients in small portions. Foods such as eggs, dairy products, avocados, vegetable oils and dried fruit can be added to dishes to increase calorie intake without weighing down digestion. In addition, protein- and calorie-rich oral food supplements, prescribed by a dietician, can be useful to support the patient's nutritional status.

## Optimizing meal conditions

As well as the composition of meals, the environment and conditions in which they are eaten play an important role for dyspneic patients. It is advisable to prepare a calm, comfortable environment, where the patient can concentrate on eating without being stressed by shortness of breath.

### Adapting your posture

The **posture** adopted during meals is essential to promote more efficient breathing. The patient should be **seated in a semi-seated**

**position**, with the torso tilted slightly forward, which frees the diaphragm and improves lung capacity during digestion. Eating in a supine or slumped position can compress the abdomen and further reduce respiratory capacity, making eating uncomfortable.

The patient should also be encouraged to **eat slowly**, taking small bites and taking the time to chew each food thoroughly. This reduces the sensation of breathlessness during a meal, and avoids swallowing too quickly, which can lead to choking or false routes.

## Promoting hydration

**Maintaining good hydration** is crucial in patients suffering from dyspnea, as hydration helps to thin bronchial secretions, making breathing easier. Patients should be encouraged to drink small amounts of fluid throughout the day, avoiding drinking large quantities all at once, which could cause a feeling of heaviness. **Warm drinks**, such as herbal teas or lukewarm water, can also help soothe the throat and ease breathing.

- Monitoring the risk of a false route in fatigued patients

**Monitoring the risk of a false route** in fatigued patients is a crucial aspect of care, particularly in those with muscular weakness, swallowing disorders (dysphagia) or respiratory pathologies. A false route occurs when food, liquids or secretions pass into the respiratory tract instead of the esophagus, which can lead to **asphyxia**, serious **lung infections** such as inhalation pneumonia, or even death in the most severe cases. Debilitated patients, whether bedridden, post-operative or chronically ill, are particularly at risk, as physical fatigue and reduced alertness impair their ability to swallow properly. Constant vigilance and appropriate preventive measures are therefore necessary to minimize these risks.

## Causes and mechanisms of false routes

**False routes** occur when the airway's protective mechanism - in particular, the closure of the epiglottis, which blocks the entrance to the larynx during swallowing - fails to function properly. This phenomenon can be exacerbated by **general fatigue, muscular weakness** or neurological disorders that impair coordination between breathing and swallowing. Patients who are fatigued, bedridden or recovering from respiratory pathology, such as pneumonia or COPD exacerbation, often present an increased risk of false swallowing, as their ability to swallow is compromised by their exhaustion and increased need to breathe rapidly.

**Muscle fatigue**, particularly of the neck and pharynx muscles, reduces swallowing efficiency, which can lead to the involuntary passage of food or liquids into the airways. In addition, **general fatigue** can impair patient alertness and coordination of respiratory movements, making it more difficult to anticipate when they need to swallow. Elderly patients or those with chronic illnesses, who are often physically weakened, are particularly vulnerable to this type of complication.

## Signs of risk of false route

**Monitoring for early signs** of a false route is essential to intervene quickly and avoid serious complications. Several **clinical signs** may indicate an increased risk or occurrence of a false route in a patient:

- **Frequent coughing** during or after meals: A reflex cough is often a warning signal that some food or liquid has entered the respiratory tract. This protective reflex attempts to clear the aspirated material, but a persistent cough should be monitored closely, as it may indicate a false route.

- **Change of voice** after swallowing: If the patient's voice becomes hoarse or muffled after eating or drinking, this may indicate that food residues or liquids have passed into the airways, disturbing the vocal cords. This suggests that swallowing is not complete or efficient.

- **Sudden shortness of breath**: A patient showing signs of respiratory distress or sudden shortness of breath during meals may have inhaled food or liquids, disrupting the airway. This must be managed immediately to avoid asphyxia or lung infection.

- **Refusal to eat** or **reduced appetite**: Patients who have experienced false-route episodes may develop **anxiety** or **fear** about eating, leading them to refuse to eat or reduce their food intake for fear of further complications. This behavior must be taken into account when adapting diet and reinforcing monitoring.

## Preventing false routes: appropriate measures

To reduce the risk of false swallowing in fatigued patients, a number of preventive measures need to be put in place. Adaptation of feeding, posture and monitoring techniques is crucial to ensure safe and efficient swallowing.

### Adapting the texture of food and the consistency of liquids

Patients with swallowing difficulties need a diet adapted to their swallowing ability. **Solid, dry** foods such as bread, cookies or meat can be difficult to chew and swallow, increasing the risk of a false route. It is therefore preferable to give preference to **soft-textured** or **blended foods**, such as purées, compotes, thick soups and chopped dishes. These foods slide more easily down the esophagus, reducing the muscular effort required to swallow.

Similarly, **fluids that are too thin** can be difficult for tired patients to control. Thickened liquids, such as juices enriched with thickening agents, pass more slowly down the throat and are therefore easier to swallow safely. The **dietician** and **speech**

**therapist** can work together to adapt the texture of meals and drinks to the patient's individual needs.

### Improving posture during meals

The patient's **posture** during meals plays a vital role in preventing false swallowing. Bedridden or debilitated patients should be placed in a **seated or semi-seated** position, with the torso inclined at around 45 degrees, to facilitate swallowing. This posture helps maintain **optimal alignment of** the head and neck, reducing the risk of food or liquids passing into the airways. Meals eaten in a recumbent position considerably increase the risk of a false route, as gravity favors the passage of the food bolus into the airways.

It is also advisable to ensure that the patient eats in a calm, stress-free environment, and to encourage him to **take his time** swallowing, by eating slowly and taking small bites or sips. Discreet but attentive monitoring during the meal enables any signs of difficulty to be detected immediately.

### Monitoring after meals

Even after meals, vigilance is essential. It's advisable to keep the patient in a **sitting** position **for at least 30 minutes** after eating or drinking, to reduce the risk of food residues rising up the throat or being aspirated into the airways. This position also helps prevent gastro-oesophageal reflux, which can aggravate the risk of food inhalation.

### Stimulating swallowing

In some patients with fatigue or neurological disorders, swallowing stimulation may be compromised. **Swallowing exercises**, often supervised by a **speech therapist**, can help strengthen throat muscles and improve coordination between breathing and swallowing. These exercises often involve working on simple but repetitive gestures that help the patient to better control swallowing movements and avoid false routes.

## Active monitoring for signs of complications

Despite all preventive measures, it is possible for a false route to occur. It is therefore essential to actively monitor for any signs of **complications** that may result from aspiration of food or fluids, such as the development of **inhalation pneumonia**. Symptoms to watch out for include **sudden fever**, **productive cough**, **increased dyspnoea**, and **chest pain**. If lung infection is suspected, medical evaluation and further tests (such as a chest X-ray) should be carried out to confirm the diagnosis and initiate antibiotic treatment if necessary.

# Chapter 5

# Oxygen therapy and respiratory care

- **The different types of oxygen therapy**
  - Low-flow oxygen, high-flow oxygen, nasal cannula, oxygen mask

**Oxygen** administration is an essential component of respiratory care, designed to correct **hypoxemia**, i.e. a lack of oxygen in the blood. Oxygen therapy helps maintain adequate oxygenation levels to support vital organ and tissue functions, particularly in patients suffering from respiratory pathologies such as **COPD, pneumonia, acute respiratory failure**, or following thoracic surgery. Depending on the severity of hypoxemia, the patient's condition and needs, oxygen can be administered at **low flow, high flow**, and via various devices such as **nasal cannula** or **oxygen mask**.

## Low-flow oxygen

**Low-flow oxygen** is commonly used for patients who require additional oxygen, but whose needs remain moderate. Typically, oxygen is administered at a flow rate of **1 to 6 liters per minute (L/min)**, increasing the fraction of inspired oxygen (FiO2) while maintaining patient comfort. This type of oxygen therapy is often used in situations where hypoxia is mild to moderate, for example in patients with stable COPD or those requiring home respiratory support.

Low-flow oxygen is often administered via **nasal** cannula, a simple, comfortable device that delivers oxygen directly into the patient's nostrils. This type of administration allows the patient to speak, eat and drink while receiving oxygen, making it a preferred choice for prolonged use, particularly in home care.

The disadvantage of this system is that, as the oxygen flow is relatively low, it may not be sufficient for patients with higher oxygen requirements. What's more, an oxygen flow of over 4 L/min via nasal cannula can cause a **sensation of dryness** and irritation in the nostrils, sometimes necessitating the addition of a **humidification** system to maintain patient comfort.

114

# High-flow oxygen

**High-flow oxygen** is intended for patients with higher oxygen requirements, generally in situations of **acute respiratory failure, respiratory distress** or severe hypoxia. This type of administration delivers oxygen flows in excess of **15 liters per minute**, with a higher oxygen concentration (FiO2 close to 100% in some cases). High-flow oxygen is essential for patients who are unable to maintain adequate oxygen saturation with low flow rates or non-invasive devices.

High-flow oxygen therapy is often administered via **an oxygen mask** or more advanced devices such as **high-flow nasal catheters.** Face masks can deliver oxygen flows of up to **10 to 15 liters per minute,** and are used in more acute settings, such as intensive care units or emergency departments. The **non-rebreathing mask**, a type of high-flow mask equipped with a reservoir and one-way valves, delivers very high concentrations of oxygen, while preventing the patient from rebreathing exhaled air, which is essential in cases of severe desaturation.

This type of oxygen administration can be uncomfortable for the patient over the long term, due to the high airflow and prolonged wearing of the mask. However, it is essential for stabilizing severely hypoxemic patients while awaiting other interventions, such as non-invasive ventilation (NIV) or intubation.

# Nasal goggles

**Nasal cannulas** are one of the most widely used devices for low-flow oxygen administration. They consist of two small probes inserted into the nostrils, linked to a tube connected to an oxygen source. This system is appreciated for its **simplicity** and **comfort,** allowing the patient to move, speak, eat and drink without interruption.

The nasal cannula delivers an oxygen flow rate of **1 to 6 L/min,** sufficient to meet the needs of many patients with mild to moderate hypoxemia. Inspired oxygen concentration varies with flow rate, with an approximate 4% increase in FiO2 per liter of oxygen delivered, reaching a maximum of around 44% with a flow rate of 6 L/min.

Although practical, nasal cannulae are not suitable for patients requiring high oxygen concentrations, as the flow rate they can deliver is limited. What's more, they can cause **discomfort** in the nostrils, particularly when oxygen is delivered at higher flow rates. In such cases, it is often advisable to add a **humidification** system to prevent dryness of the nasal mucosa.

## Oxygen mask

The **oxygen mask** is a device with greater coverage than nasal cannula, used to deliver oxygen at **higher concentrations** and **higher flow rates**. It is generally made of flexible plastic and covers the nose and mouth, ensuring more even oxygen delivery. This device is particularly useful when oxygen requirements are higher, exceeding what nasal cannula can provide.

There are several types of oxygen masks:

- **Single mask**: delivers oxygen at a flow rate of **5 to 10 L/ min**, with a FiO2 of between **40% and 60%**. The single mask is used in situations of moderate hypoxemia, when nasal cannula are not sufficient, but the patient's situation does not require a very high oxygen supply.

- **High-concentration mask with reservoir**: Also known as a **non-rebreather mask**, it features a reservoir bag that fills with oxygen and allows the patient to inhale pure oxygen, without rebreathing exhaled air. This mask is capable of delivering oxygen flows of up to **15 L/min**, with a FiO2 close to **100%**, which is essential for patients in severe respiratory distress.

- **Venturi mask**: This mask is used to deliver oxygen at a precise concentration. It is equipped with color-coded valves, each corresponding to a specific flow rate and oxygen concentration. The Venturi mask is ideal for patients requiring **controlled FiO2**, such as those suffering from COPD, where it is crucial to avoid hyperoxia while treating hypoxemia.

The disadvantage of the oxygen mask is that it can be **less comfortable** for the patient than nasal cannula, especially when worn for long periods. It can also make communication more difficult and interfere with activities such as eating and drinking.

- The caregiver's role in installation and monitoring

**The caregiver's role** in patient care is fundamental to ensuring comfort, safety and quality of care. Whether in the hospital or at home, the nursing auxiliary is a pillar of daily patient care, working closely with the medical team and paying attention to the smallest details. They play a decisive role in **setting up** and **monitoring** patients, from correct positioning to the use of medical devices and the prevention of complications. This role encompasses a variety of tasks, from physical and psychological support to the implementation of specific technical interventions, always with the patient's well-being in mind.

## Settling the patient: essential basic care

Patient positioning is a fundamental act which, although it may seem simple, has a significant impact on **comfort, prevention of complications** and **quality of care**. Every step in the installation process must be carefully considered, adapted to the patient's condition, and always carried out with gentleness and respect.

One of the caregiver's first tasks is to help the patient settle in comfortably and safely. This starts with **setting up the bedding**, adjusting sheets and pillows to provide adequate support, while avoiding the formation of folds that could cause discomfort or rubbing, especially in bedridden patients. Bed position should be changed regularly to avoid **pressure sores** and other complications associated with prolonged immobility, notably by stimulating **blood circulation** and relieving pressure points.

The caregiver's role is also essential in the **ergonomic positioning of** patients, especially those suffering from respiratory diseases. In collaboration with the nurse or doctor, the caregiver helps to position the patient correctly to facilitate breathing, for example by placing the patient in a **semi-seated position** (Fowler's position) to relieve pressure on the diaphragm and allow better lung expansion.

This is particularly important for patients undergoing **oxygen therapy** or requiring medical devices. The caregiver ensures that **nasal cannula**, **oxygen masks** or other devices are correctly positioned, ensuring **optimal oxygen flow** without discomfort or leakage. He or she adjusts tubing to avoid pinching, and ensures that devices are comfortably positioned so as not to irritate the patient's skin, while preventing wires and tubes from becoming obstacles or sources of discomfort.

## Continuous monitoring: vigilance and responsiveness

**Monitoring** is one of the most crucial aspects of a caregiver's work. Monitoring is both **visual** and **clinical**, and is based on careful listening to the patient. It must be continuous, so that any sign of deterioration or complication can be rapidly detected. Warning signs may be subtle, but constant vigilance enables rapid intervention and the prevention of more serious situations.

One element of monitoring is observing the patient's **breathing**, particularly in those with respiratory pathologies. The caregiver is often the first to notice changes in respiratory rate, signs of **dyspnea** or excessive use of **accessory respiratory muscles**. If a patient on oxygen therapy shows a **drop in oxygen saturation** or worsening dyspnea, the caregiver can alert the nursing team to quickly adjust the oxygen flow or consider other interventions.

At the same time, the caregiver must be attentive to more general **physical parameters**, such as **skin color** (pallor, cyanosis), **body temperature**, and the appearance of cold sweats, which may indicate signs of respiratory or circulatory distress. Regular monitoring of vital signs (respiratory rate, heart rate, oxygen saturation) is an integral part of this surveillance.

In addition, the caregiver monitors the **medical devices** in place. If **nasal cannula** or **oxygen mask are** used, he or she must check that these devices are working properly, that there are no oxygen disconnections or leaks, and that the patient is tolerating them well. Furthermore, in cases where more complex respiratory assistance devices are used (such as non-invasive ventilation or oxygen concentrators), he assists with their basic maintenance, ensuring that they are clean, properly adjusted and in good working order.

## Preventing complications: an active role

Caregivers play an active role in **preventing complications** linked to immobility or medical devices. In the case of bedridden patients, they are constantly on the lookout to prevent the development of **pressure sores**. This involves not only regular repositioning of the patient to avoid pressure points, but also frequent inspection of at-risk areas, such as the heels, sacrum and elbows, for early detection of redness or irritation. Applying moisturizing or protective creams to at-risk areas is also part of preventive care.

For patients on **oxygen therapy**, the caregiver must also ensure that the patient's skin is not irritated by **oxygen delivery devices**. Nasal goggles can cause nostril irritation or dryness, while masks can create pressure points or rubbing on the face. In such cases, the caregiver applies appropriate skin care products, such as moisturizing creams or protective pads, to prevent irritation and ensure greater patient comfort.

## Psychological and relational support

As well as providing technical and physical care, the nursing auxiliary has a central role to play in providing **psychological support** to the patient. They are often on the front line in building a relationship of **trust** with patients, encouraging and reassuring them, particularly when they are distressed by their illness or respiratory situation. This caring presence helps patients feel listened to and supported, while contributing to their general well-being.

The caregiver can also play an essential role in **patient** and family **education**, especially for patients who need to return home with oxygen therapy or other devices. They explain how to use the devices, how to prevent complications, and how to alert the patient if a problem arises. This educational role promotes patient autonomy while reducing the risk of misuse of medical devices.

- **Monitoring the side effects of oxygen therapy**
  - Dry mouth, nasal lesions

**Dry mouth** and **nasal lesions** are frequent complications in patients undergoing prolonged oxygen therapy or suffering from chronic respiratory pathologies. Although these discomforts may seem minor, they can significantly affect the comfort and well-being of patients, particularly those undergoing high-flow oxygen treatment or using devices such as **nasal cannula** or **oxygen masks**. Their management requires a careful, personalized approach, to prevent pain, improve quality of life and avoid possible secondary complications.

# Dry mouth: causes and impacts

**Dry mouth**, or **xerostomia**, is a common side effect in patients undergoing oxygen therapy, particularly when oxygen is administered via **nasal cannula** or high-flow **mask**. The dry, cold air delivered by these devices can reduce the natural moisture content of the mouth and mucous membranes, resulting in an uncomfortable sensation of dry mouth. This dryness can also result from certain drug treatments (such as bronchodilators or antihistamines) or from mouth breathing, common in patients suffering from **dyspnea** or **nasal congestion**.

Dry mouth may seem harmless, but it can have significant consequences for the patient. In addition to the discomfort it generates, it can lead to **difficulty in speaking, dysphagia** (difficulty in swallowing), and sometimes an alteration in the taste of food, reducing the patient's appetite. It also increases the risk of developing **oral infections**, such as **candidiasis** (yeast infection), and lesions of the gums or tongue. A dry mouth is also more vulnerable to **lesions** and **ulcerations**, which can become hotbeds of infection.

# Nasal lesions: causes and risks

**Nasal lesions** are another common side effect in patients receiving oxygen via **nasal cannula or oxygen mask**. Prolonged administration of dry, concentrated oxygen can irritate the nasal mucosa, leading to excessive **dryness, crusting** and sometimes **bleeding** (epistaxis). Nasal goggles can also cause continuous **rubbing of** the skin around the nostrils, nose and behind the ears, leading to skin irritation and superficial lesions.

These nasal lesions, although often superficial, can become painful, impede oxygen delivery and increase the risk of infection. Nasal **crusting** and **bleeding** can also complicate nasal breathing, forcing patients to breathe through the mouth, which in turn aggravates dry mouth.

121

## Prevention and management measures

To prevent and alleviate **dry mouth** and **nasal lesions**, it's essential to adopt a proactive approach, combining simple hydration measures with appropriate local care. These measures not only improve patient comfort, but also prevent more serious complications, such as infection or ulceration.

### Mucous membrane hydration

One of the first steps in preventing dry mouth is to ensure that patients are well **hydrated**. It's important to encourage patients to drink small amounts of water regularly throughout the day, to maintain adequate mucosal hydration. **Frequent sips** of water, or the use of **crushed ice** to moisten the mouth without weighing down the stomach, are simple and effective measures.

For patients with severe dry mouth, **salivary substitutes** or moisturizing **sprays specially** designed to maintain moisture in the mouth can be used. These products, available as gels or solutions, quickly relieve the sensation of dry mouth and protect mucous membranes from irritation. In addition, sugar-free **chewing gums** or lozenges can stimulate natural saliva production, helping to maintain sufficient oral moisture.

### Oxygen humidification

To prevent nasal and oral dryness caused by the administration of dry oxygen, it is advisable to add a **humidification system** to the oxygen, especially when high flow rates are used. These humidifiers warm and humidify the administered air, reducing the drying effect of oxygen on mucous membranes.

Whether in the hospital or at home, the caregiver ensures that these humidification systems are correctly installed and operating efficiently. Regular monitoring of device cleanliness is also essential to prevent the proliferation of bacteria or fungi in humidifiers, which could lead to respiratory infections.

### Local care of nasal lesions

To prevent and treat **nasal lesions**, it's important to regularly inspect the skin around the nostrils and the nasal mucosa for irritation, redness or crusting. In the event of dryness or nasal crusting, the application of **saline solutions** or seawater-based sprays can help moisturize mucous membranes and remove crusts without further irritating tissues.

**Vaseline-based moisturizers** or **balms** can also be applied around the nostrils to protect the skin from rubbing against the nasal cannula. However, the use of petroleum-based products in the nasal passages should be limited in patients undergoing oxygen therapy, as they can increase the risk of inhalation of oily particles, which can lead to pulmonary complications. It is therefore preferable to use specific, non-greasy **moisturizing creams** to avoid this risk.

If nasal lesions are more extensive, or if **bleeding** occurs frequently, it's advisable to notify your doctor. He or she may prescribe healing or antiseptic ointments to promote healing and prevent secondary infection.

## Patient follow-up and education

The caregiver plays a key role in **monitoring** and **preventing** these complications, by making patients aware of the importance of hydration and teaching them how to care for their skin and mucous membranes. It's crucial that patients on prolonged oxygen therapy are aware of the signs to watch out for, such as excessive dryness, crusting or pain, and know how to react.

The caregiver also regularly inspects oxygen delivery devices, adjusting **nasal cannula** to prevent rubbing, and checking that oxygen humidification is correctly applied. This preventive monitoring helps to limit the discomfort associated with oxygen therapy and improve patients' quality of life.

◦     Monitor for signs of hyperoxia or hypoxia

**Monitoring for signs of hyperoxia** (excess oxygen in the blood) and **hypoxia** (deficiency of oxygen in the blood) is essential in the management of patients undergoing oxygen therapy or suffering from respiratory pathologies. Maintaining an optimal balance in oxygen delivery is crucial to avoid serious complications. Oxygen therapy mismanagement can lead to imbalances, with deleterious effects on the patient's organs and tissues. Vigilance on the part of caregivers, and particularly nursing assistants, is essential to prevent and detect such imbalances at an early stage.

## Understanding hypoxia

**Hypoxia** occurs when tissues do not receive sufficient oxygen to perform their vital functions. It may be due to respiratory failure, airway obstruction, heart disease or blood circulation disorders. Untreated hypoxia can rapidly lead to irreversible organ damage and, in the most severe cases, multiple organ failure.

The clinical signs of hypoxia vary according to its severity, but the most common include:

- **Dyspnea**: Difficulty in breathing or shortness of breath is often one of the first signs of hypoxia. The patient may breathe faster or more deeply in an attempt to compensate for the lack of oxygen.

- **Cyanosis**: **Cyanosis** is a bluish discoloration of the skin and mucous membranes, particularly around the lips, nails and extremities. It indicates severe hypoxia, when blood oxygen saturation is below 85%.

- **Tachycardia**: In response to hypoxia, the heart tries to compensate by beating faster, in order to increase oxygen delivery to vital organs. This results in an increase in heart rate, which can be observed by monitoring vital signs.

- **Confusion or agitation**: Cerebral hypoxia, i.e. lack of oxygen to the brain, can cause neurological symptoms such as confusion, agitation or irritability. In some patients, this may manifest as excessive sleepiness or difficulty concentrating.

- **Altered state of consciousness**: In severe forms of hypoxia, the patient may lose consciousness or lapse into **stupor** or **coma**, signaling an imminent risk to survival.

Caregivers need to be alert to these signs in their daily monitoring, particularly in patients on oxygen therapy or with a history of respiratory illness. Regular monitoring of **oxygen saturation (SpO2)** with a pulse oximeter helps to keep track of oxygen levels in the blood. If saturation falls below **90%**, this should alert the caregiver and lead to a rapid reassessment of oxygenation treatment.

## Understanding hyperoxia

**Hyperoxia**, on the other hand, is less well known than hypoxia, but also presents serious risks, particularly in patients suffering from chronic respiratory diseases such as **COPD**. Hyperoxia occurs when patients receive too much oxygen in relation to their physiological needs. Excess oxygen can disrupt respiratory regulation mechanisms, cause carbon dioxide retention (hypercapnia) and lead to lung and central nervous system damage. This is particularly dangerous in COPD patients, where high oxygen concentrations can reduce respiratory drive and worsen respiratory failure.

Clinical signs of hyperoxia may include:

- **Headaches**: Headaches can be an early sign of hyperoxia, caused by carbon dioxide retention in the blood. The patient may complain of diffuse pain or more intense migraines.

- **Excessive drowsiness**: **Hypoventilation** may occur in hyperoxic patients, leading to increased carbon dioxide levels in the blood. This can lead to unusual drowsiness, or even lethargy.

- **Nausea**: Gastrointestinal disorders such as nausea or vomiting may occur in the event of excess oxygen, particularly when the inspired oxygen concentration is too high.

- **Deterioration of respiratory function**: In severe cases, hyperoxia can lead to respiratory decompensation, with a paradoxical increase in dyspnea or signs of respiratory fatigue. The patient may begin to breathe more shallowly or more slowly, indicating respiratory muscle exhaustion.

- **Reddening of the skin**: In some cases, reddening of the skin may occur, particularly on the face, in response to an overdose of oxygen.

Caregivers need to be particularly vigilant in patients at high risk of hyperoxia, such as those with COPD or chronic respiratory failure, where **excessive oxygen administration** can worsen their condition. It is crucial to closely monitor **oxygen saturation** and ensure that levels do not exceed prescribed thresholds. For example, in COPD patients, excessive **FiO2** )fraction of inspired oxygen) above 92% can lead to adverse effects.

## Monitoring and adjusting oxygen therapy

One of the caregiver's major roles is to monitor the patient's **vital parameters** regularly and carefully, in order to detect any alterations indicative of hypoxia or hyperoxia. The use of a **pulse oximeter enables oxygen saturation (SpO2)** to be monitored in real time, while **respiratory rate** and **heart rate** can provide additional clues to the patient's clinical condition. Normal oxygen saturation should be maintained between **95 and 100%** in a healthy patient, while in a COPD patient, SpO2 should be maintained between **88 and 92%** to avoid the risk of hyperoxia.

In addition to vital vitals, the caregiver must be attentive to the patient's **physical signs** and **behavioral symptoms**, such as changes in consciousness, cyanosis, agitation or drowsiness. Regular communication with the patient is essential to identify subtle symptoms of discomfort, whether headaches or shortness of breath.

If hypoxia or hyperoxia is suspected, the caregiver must **immediately inform the medical team** to adjust oxygen therapy. If **hypoxia** is confirmed, the oxygen flow rate can be increased according to the medical prescription to rapidly correct saturation. If **hyperoxia** is detected, the oxygen supply needs to be reduced, while closely monitoring for signs of respiratory deterioration.

- **Bronchial clearance techniques**

  ○ Help with secretion mobilization (controlled cough, physiotherapy techniques)

**Assisting with secretion mobilization** is a fundamental aspect of pulmonary care, particularly in patients suffering from chronic respiratory diseases such as **COPD, cystic fibrosis**, or during convalescence from acute lung infections such as pneumonia. These patients may have difficulty **evacuating the secretions** that build up in their airways, leading to bronchial obstruction, worsening dyspnoea and an increased risk of respiratory infections. To prevent these complications and improve patients' quality of life, it is essential to implement strategies aimed at facilitating the evacuation of secretions, through techniques such as **controlled coughing** or **respiratory physiotherapy exercises**.

# The importance of mobilizing secretions

The accumulation of **bronchial secretions** is a frequent problem in patients with chronic or acute respiratory pathologies. These secretions, composed of mucus and cellular debris, can obstruct the airways and reduce the efficiency of gas exchange in the lungs. When secretions stagnate in the bronchial tubes, they become a breeding ground for infection, leading to a worsening of the patient's respiratory condition and an increased risk of **pneumonia**.

Facilitating the mobilization and evacuation of secretions is therefore essential to prevent airway obstruction and improve lung function. This helps to **clear bronchial tubes**, reduce breathlessness and promote better oxygenation. The nursing auxiliary plays a central role in implementing these techniques, guiding and accompanying the patient through the various methods of secretion mobilization.

## Controlled coughing

**Controlled coughing** is one of the simplest and most effective ways to help patients clear secretions from the respiratory tract. Unlike spontaneous coughing, which can be exhausting and ineffective, controlled coughing is a structured technique that expels mucus without causing excessive fatigue or respiratory discomfort.

The caregiver can teach the **controlled cough technique** to the patient in several steps:

1. **Position the patient correctly**: The patient should be in a seated position, leaning slightly forward, with feet firmly planted on the floor and arms resting on the thighs. This position maximizes the efficiency of the respiratory muscles and frees up the diaphragm.

2. **Take a deep breath**: The patient should inhale deeply, trying to fill the lungs with air. This deep inhalation helps ventilate the bronchial tubes, facilitating the mobilization of mucus into the upper respiratory tract.

3. **Close the glottis and contract the abdominal muscles**: Before expelling air, the patient should close the glottis (by slightly squeezing the throat) and contract the abdominal muscles. This creates pressure in the airways, helping to expel mucus.

4. **Expel air with a short, dry cough**: The patient then exhales rapidly, producing a short, dry cough without excessive force. This method effectively expels mucus without causing exhaustion or respiratory discomfort.

Controlled coughing should be repeated several times, with pauses between each cough to avoid fatigue. The caregiver must be attentive to the patient's comfort, ensuring that he or she does not feel pain or exhaustion during the exercise.

## Respiratory physiotherapy techniques

**Respiratory physiotherapy** is another crucial method for helping to mobilize secretions. It relies on specific techniques to clear the airways, improve respiratory function and reduce mucus build-up. These techniques are often taught by **specialized physiotherapists**, but the caregiver plays a key role in accompanying the patient through these exercises, particularly at home or in hospital.

**Postural drainage**

**Postural drainage** is a technique designed to use gravity to facilitate the evacuation of secretions from the deepest areas of the lungs. It involves positioning the patient so that the lung segments containing secretions are oriented upwards, allowing mucus to flow towards the main bronchi, from where it can be expelled by coughing.

Postural drainage is generally performed in the **supine position** or with the patient inclined at different angles, depending on the location of secretions. For example, if mucus accumulates in the lower lobes of the lungs, the patient will be tilted with the head downwards to favor gravity. This positioning can be performed several times a day, and is often accompanied by chest percussion to enhance drainage efficiency.

**Thoracic percussion**

**Thoracic percussion**, also known as **clapping**, is a technique that involves gently tapping the patient's ribcage with cupped hands. This creates a vibration that helps loosen mucus from the bronchial walls, facilitating its expulsion. This technique is often used in combination with postural drainage to improve secretion mobilization.

Caregivers, trained in this technique, must ensure that percussion is gentle and rhythmic, avoiding any pain or discomfort for the patient. Clapping should be applied to areas of the thorax corresponding to congested lobes, and may be followed by a controlled coughing session to expel mobilized secretions.

**Forced exhalation techniques**

**Forced exhalation techniques**, such as **huffing**, are also effective in clearing the airways. **Huffing** is a rapid, powerful exhalation, performed without blocking the glottis, which mobilizes secretions from the distal bronchi to the upper airways. Unlike coughing, huffing is less tiring and reduces the risk of bronchial spasm.

To **huff**, the patient inhales deeply, then exhales rapidly with the mouth open, producing a sound similar to a "ha". This technique is particularly useful for patients suffering from bronchial obstruction, as it clears secretions without causing excessive airway contraction.

## Hydration and humidification

Helping to mobilize secretions is not limited to physical techniques. **Good hydration** is essential to liquefy mucus and facilitate its expulsion. Patients should be encouraged to drink enough water throughout the day to prevent secretions from becoming too thick and difficult to eliminate.

In addition, the use of air **humidification** devices, such as oxygen humidifiers for patients on oxygen therapy, can help maintain airway moisture and prevent the formation of thick, sticky secretions.

◦   Use of bronchial suction and nebulizer devices

**Bronchial suction** and **nebulization devices** are widely used in pulmonology, particularly for patients with severe respiratory difficulties or excessive accumulation of bronchial secretions. Both devices help improve respiratory function, prevent airway obstruction and optimize drug delivery. The role of the caregiver is essential in the use and monitoring of these devices, to ensure their smooth operation and patient comfort.

## Bronchial suction: clearing the airways

**Bronchial suctioning** is a technique used to remove secretions from the airways when the patient is unable to evacuate them on his or her own, either due to muscular weakness, chronic respiratory disease, or after intubation or tracheostomy. The accumulation of secretions, particularly in bedridden or mechanically ventilated patients, can lead to bronchial obstruction, aggravate breathlessness and increase the risk of pulmonary infection, such as inhalation pneumonia.

The principle of bronchial suctioning is to use a **suction device** that generates negative pressure to remove accumulated secretions from the airways. This procedure is generally performed using a **flexible catheter**, inserted into the airways via the nose, mouth or tracheostomy.

**Bronchial aspiration procedure**

Bronchial aspiration must be performed with care to minimize the risk of mucosal trauma and preserve patient comfort. Here are the main steps in the procedure:

1. **Preparing the equipment**: The caregiver prepares all the necessary equipment, including a functional suction device, a sterile catheter, gloves and saline solution if required. Adjustment of the device is essential to avoid over-aggressive suctioning, which could damage bronchial tissue.

2. **Ensure proper oxygenation**: Before starting suctioning, it is important to ensure that the patient is properly oxygenated. In patients on oxygen therapy, it may be necessary to temporarily increase the oxygen flow to compensate for the brief interruption of breathing during aspiration.

3. **Catheter insertion**: The caregiver gently inserts the catheter into the airway until it reaches the secretions. It is crucial to be attentive to the patient's reactions, and to avoid inserting the catheter too deeply, in order to limit coughing or vomiting reflexes.

4. **Aspiration of secretions**: By activating the device, aspiration is performed for a few seconds while the catheter is slowly withdrawn. This technique effectively collects secretions without damaging the mucous membranes. Suction must be interrupted between each passage to allow the patient to recover.

5. **Patient monitoring**: Throughout the procedure, the caregiver must monitor the patient's **vital signs**, such as oxygen saturation, heart rate and respiratory rate. Any deterioration in the patient's condition (cyanosis, bradycardia, shortness of breath) should be reported immediately.

**Indications and precautions**

Bronchial aspiration is indicated for patients unable to cough up secretions. It is common in **mechanically ventilated** patients, tracheostomized patients and those suffering from neuromuscular diseases. However, it must be performed with care, as too frequent or too aggressive suctioning can lead to mucosal irritation, bleeding or infection.

The caregiver plays an essential role in assessing the **need for suctioning** and in preventing associated complications. After the procedure, he or she keeps the airways moist and hydrates the patient to promote better mobilization of secretions.

# Nebulization: aerosolized drug delivery

**Nebulization** is a technique used to administer drugs in aerosol form directly into the respiratory tract. It is commonly used in patients suffering from **bronchospasm** (in asthma or COPD), to thin secretions, or to deliver antibiotics in the event of lung infection. Unlike bronchial aspiration, whose aim is to clear the airways, nebulization is designed to **treat** the respiratory tract by administering medication in mist form.

Nebulizers consist of a **nebulizer**, which converts liquid medication into fine particles, and a **face mask** or **mouthpiece** through which the patient inhales the treatment. Medications frequently administered by nebulization include **bronchodilators** (to open airways), **mucolytics** (to thin mucus) and corticosteroids (to reduce inflammation).

**Nebulization procedure**

Nebulization is a simple procedure that can be carried out at home or in hospital. Here are the key steps to successful nebulization:

1. **Medication preparation**: The caregiver prepares the prescribed drug solution according to the doctor's recommendations. It may be a ready-to-use solution or a mixture of several drugs.

2. **Setting up the device**: The nebulizer is connected to an air compressor, which transforms the liquid solution into an aerosol. A face mask or mouthpiece is then placed over the patient's face, covering the mouth and nose to ensure optimum inhalation.

3. **Inhalation supervision**: The patient inhales the aerosol particles slowly and deeply over a period of approximately 10 to 15 minutes. The caregiver should encourage the patient to breathe calmly, ensuring that the inhalation is carried out correctly. For children or elderly patients, the mask may be more comfortable than the mouthpiece.

4. **Cleaning the device**: After each use, it is crucial to clean the nebulizer thoroughly to avoid infections. The caregiver must ensure that the device is well maintained and ready for the next nebulization session.

## Indications and follow-up

Nebulization is often prescribed for patients suffering from **asthma**, **COPD** or other obstructive pathologies. It enables rapid administration of bronchodilator or anti-inflammatory drugs, which act directly on the bronchial tubes, reducing inflammation and improving airflow. It is also used in patients with thick secretions that are difficult to expectorate, as certain mucolytics can be administered in aerosol form to thin mucus.

During and after nebulization, the caregiver monitors the effectiveness of the treatment by observing the patient's **respiratory rate, oxygen saturation** and **tolerance**. It's also important to watch out for any drug side effects, such as **tachycardia** or tremors, especially after inhalation of bronchodilators like salbutamol.

# Chapter 6

# Medical device management in pulmonology

- **Introduction to respiratory equipment and machines**
  - ◦ Ventilators, CPAP, BiPAP machines

**Ventilators**, **CPAP** and **BiPAP** machines are essential devices in the management of patients suffering from **respiratory distress**, **sleep apnea,** or chronic diseases such as **COPD** or **respiratory failure**. These devices help maintain efficient breathing in patients who have difficulty breathing spontaneously or maintaining adequate ventilation. Their use is based on specific principles designed to improve oxygenation and support respiratory effort, according to the patient's level of need. The role of caregivers, and in particular nursing assistants, is crucial in ensuring that these devices are correctly fitted, and that they are continuously monitored to guarantee their effectiveness and the patient's comfort.

## Ventilators: breathing support in acute distress

**Mechanical ventilators** are mainly used in hospitals, particularly in intensive care units, for patients who are unable to breathe independently, or who require significant ventilatory assistance. These machines can **partially or totally replace the** patient's **respiratory effort** by controlling or assisting breathing cycles (inhalation and exhalation). Ventilators are indispensable for intubated or tracheostomized patients, particularly in cases of acute respiratory distress, severe pneumonia, or during recovery from major thoracic surgery.

**Fan operation**

The **mechanical ventilator** is a complex device that regulates the pressure and volume of air or oxygen delivered to the patient's lungs. Depending on the mode of ventilation, the ventilator can either **take over** breathing **completely,** or **assist** the patient by facilitating inhalation while allowing passive exhalation.

The ventilators can operate in several modes, adapted to the specific needs of the patient:

- **Pressure-controlled ventilation**: In this mode, the device delivers a predefined air pressure to open the patient's lungs. This mode is used when lung compliance (lung elasticity) is low, as in **acute respiratory distress syndrome** (ARDS).

- **Volume-controlled ventilation**: The ventilator delivers a fixed volume of air with each inspiration, ensuring adequate ventilation even if lung pressure varies. This mode is often used in intensive care patients with severely impaired lung function.

- **Assisted-controlled ventilation**: This mode allows the patient to initiate spontaneous breathing, but the ventilator provides assistance for each inspiration, ensuring adequate volume or pressure. This mode is useful for patients undergoing ventilatory weaning.

**Monitoring and the role of caregivers**

The use of a ventilator requires **constant monitoring** to ensure that the patient is receiving adequate oxygenation and that the device is working properly. The caregiver, in collaboration with the medical team, must monitor **vital signs** such as respiratory rate, oxygen saturation (SpO2) and blood pressure, as well as regularly checking the condition of the patient's airways (endotracheal tube, tracheostomy). Any ventilator alarms, whether pressure or volume changes, or technical anomalies, must be dealt with immediately to avoid serious complications.

# CPAP: continuous positive airway pressure

**CPAP** (Continuous Positive Airway Pressure) is a machine used to keep the airways open by providing a constant flow of pressurized air into the lungs. Unlike mechanical ventilators, CPAP does not directly assist the respiratory process; it provides a constant air pressure that prevents **airway collapse**, which is particularly useful in patients suffering from **obstructive sleep apnea** or **mild to moderate respiratory insufficiency**.

## Using CPAP

CPAP is commonly used in patients suffering from sleep apnea, a condition in which the upper airway collapses during sleep, interrupting breathing. The machine delivers a continuous flow of air through a **mask** worn over the nose or mouth, preventing airway obstruction during the night. This airflow maintains a constant pressure, known as **positive pressure**, which keeps the airways open, enabling the patient to breathe normally during sleep.

CPAP is also used in more acute settings, such as in patients suffering from **COPD** or **congestive heart failure**, where it helps reduce **dyspnea** by increasing lung capacity and improving gas exchange.

### Monitoring and adaptation

The caregiver plays an essential role in fitting the CPAP mask and monitoring its effectiveness. The mask must fit snugly to avoid air leaks, but not too tightly to cause discomfort or skin injury. It's also important to ensure that the patient tolerates the air pressure, which can be uncomfortable at first. Monitoring vital signs, such as oxygen saturation, helps to assess whether CPAP is effective and whether adjustments are necessary.

## BiPAP: dual-level pressure ventilation

**BiPAP** (Bilevel Positive Airway Pressure), or dual-level pressure ventilation, is a machine similar to CPAP, but it offers two different pressure levels: a higher pressure during inspiration

(**IPAP**) and a lower pressure during expiration (**EPAP**). This alternation of pressures helps to facilitate inspiration while keeping the airway open during exhalation, making BiPAP more suitable for patients requiring greater respiratory assistance than that provided by CPAP.

## Using BiPAP

BiPAP is often prescribed for patients suffering from **severe COPD**, **respiratory failure** or **restrictive syndromes** where the respiratory muscles are weakened, as in neuromuscular diseases. It is also used in patients with **central sleep apnea**, where apnea is caused by a disruption in the brain's signal to breathe, rather than a physical obstruction of the airways.

The main advantage of BiPAP is that it reduces the workload on the respiratory muscles, making inspiration easier, while enabling easier exhalation with less pressure. This is particularly useful for patients who find it difficult to exhale completely, or who have severely obstructed airways.

## Patient monitoring and comfort

As with CPAP, the caregiver plays a crucial role in fitting the BiPAP mask and monitoring the patient's condition. Because of the fluctuating pressure, some patients may need time to adapt to the machine. The caregiver must ensure that the patient is comfortable and does not experience **dyspnea** or excessive discomfort during use. **Blood gas** monitoring may also be necessary to assess BiPAP effectiveness and adjust pressure levels if necessary.

  ◦  Device management skills
**Managing** respiratory **equipment** such as **ventilators**, **CPAP** and **BiPAP** machines requires a specific set of **technical** and **human skills**. These skills enable caregivers to use these devices safely and effectively, while ensuring patient comfort and well-being.

The correct use of these devices, often vital for patients in respiratory distress or suffering from chronic illnesses, relies on in-depth knowledge of their operation, individual patient needs, and monitoring and maintenance protocols. Here are the main skills needed to manage respiratory equipment.

# 1. Technical knowledge of equipment

**Mastery of the technical aspects** of ventilators, CPAP and BiPAP machines is essential to ensure effective use. This includes understanding the different ventilation modes, handling settings, and knowing the associated monitoring systems.

- **Machine operation**: Know how each machine works, including the principles of continuous positive airway pressure (CPAP) and bi-level positive airway pressure (BiPAP), as well as the ventilation modes of mechanical ventilators. This includes management of parameters such as **inspiratory pressure** (IPAP), **expiratory pressure** (EPAP), tidal volume, and alarms.

- **Adapting settings**: Understand how to adapt device settings to the patient's specific needs. For example, for a COPD patient, managing pressure levels to avoid hyperoxia or hypoxia is crucial. Knowing how to adjust pressure and flow rates according to therapeutic objectives is essential.

- **Alarm recognition**: It's vital to recognize and interpret device **alarm signals**, whether they are pressure problems, airway obstruction or circuit disconnection. Caregivers need to react quickly to correct these anomalies and ensure optimal ventilation.

- **Care and maintenance**: Ensuring that machines are properly maintained - including the cleanliness of masks, tubing, filters and water tanks in the case of humidification units - is essential to prevent infections and breakdowns.

The ability to detect signs of wear or malfunction is part of technical management.

## 2. Clinical monitoring

**Clinical monitoring** is a fundamental skill, as it enables us to assess the effectiveness of the devices and ensure that the patient is responding well to treatment.

- **Vital signs observation**: Measure and interpret the patient's vital signs, such as **oxygen saturation (SpO2)**, **respiratory rate**, **heart rate** and **blood pressure**, to ensure that the machine is maintaining adequate oxygenation. Any change in these parameters may indicate a need for machine adjustment.

- **Detecting signs of respiratory distress**: Be able to identify early signs of **respiratory distress**, such as increased dyspnea, use of accessory muscles, cyanosis or tachycardia. By monitoring clinical status, treatment can be adjusted rapidly before the situation deteriorates.

- **Knowledge of blood gases**: Understanding the results of **arterial blood gas** analyses (PaO2, PaCO2, pH) enables precise assessment of the quality of gas exchange in patients on assisted ventilation or in chronic respiratory failure. These data can be used to guide adjustments to ventilator or CPAP/BiPAP machine parameters.

## 3. Adaptability

Every patient has unique ventilation needs. The ability to adapt care as the patient's respiratory condition evolves is essential.

- **Personalized care**: adapting the device and its use to the patient's specific needs, whether for a tracheotomized patient on a ventilator or a sleep apnea sufferer using a CPAP. For example, air pressure and oxygen requirements vary according to the patient's clinical condition and pathology.

- **Management of anxious or intolerant patients**: Some patients may experience significant discomfort with CPAP/BiPAP masks or ventilators, due to air pressure or claustrophobia. The caregiver needs to be patient, adjust the mask for comfort, and provide psychological support to help adaptation.

- **Adjustment to changing clinical conditions**: Patients' respiratory conditions may change over time. It is therefore necessary to know how to adjust settings according to signs of stabilization or worsening, and to coordinate with the medical team for more extensive adjustments.

## 4. Communication with the patient and medical team

Respirator management is not just about technical skills; good communication is also essential.

- **Informing the patient**: It's crucial to **communicate clearly** with the patient about how the device works, explaining why it's needed, how it will help, and what the patient may experience during its use. This helps to reduce patient anxiety and improve cooperation.

- **Reporting anomalies**: Any abnormal observations concerning the device's efficiency or the patient's clinical condition must be immediately communicated to the care team, whether the nurse in charge or the doctor. Accurate information is essential for rapid decision-making.

- **Team coordination**: Caregivers must be able to work as part of a **multidisciplinary team**, in collaboration with doctors, nurses, physiotherapists and other healthcare professionals, to ensure optimum management of equipment and care.

## 5. Human and interpersonal skills

Finally, managing respiratory equipment requires **human skills**. Caregivers are often in the front line when it comes to reassuring patients, especially those who find it difficult to fit a ventilator or CPAP/BiPAP machine.

- **Empathy and listening**: Patients in respiratory distress can be very anxious or disoriented. The caregiver must show **compassion**, taking the time to reassure the patient and listen to his or her needs and comfort.

- **Psychological support**: prolonged use of respiratory equipment can generate stress, feelings of dependence or frustration in patients. Ongoing moral support is therefore necessary to help patients accept and adapt to their treatment.

- **Maintenance and monitoring of respiratory devices**
  - Device hygiene: infection prevention

**Respiratory device hygiene** is an essential aspect in the management of patients using devices such as **ventilators, CPAP, BiPAP**, or other respiratory assistance systems. Poor hygiene of such equipment can lead to **nosocomial infections**, such as ventilator-associated pneumonia, which increase morbidity and mortality in vulnerable patients. Infection prevention relies on rigorous hygiene management, including proper cleaning, disinfection and maintenance of devices. The nursing auxiliary plays a key role in this prevention, ensuring patient safety while keeping equipment running smoothly.

# Risks associated with respiratory devices

Respiratory devices, such as **ventilators, nasal cannula, oxygen masks, nebulizers** and **CPAP/BiPAP** systems, are in direct contact with the patient's airways. These devices can easily become vectors of contamination if strict hygiene protocols are not followed. **Bacteria, viruses** and **fungi can** lodge in tubing, masks, filters or water reservoirs, leading to serious lung infections.

The most common infections associated with these devices are **ventilation-associated pneumonia (VAP)** and upper respiratory tract infections. Patients most vulnerable to these infections are those on prolonged mechanical ventilation, the immunocompromised, and those suffering from chronic respiratory diseases such as **COPD** or **cystic fibrosis**.

## Cleaning and disinfection practices for respiratory devices

**Disinfection** and **cleaning of** respiratory devices are crucial steps in limiting the risk of contamination. These practices must be rigorously followed in both hospital and homecare environments.

### Cleaning masks and tubing

**Respiratory masks**, whether used for CPAP, BiPAP or mechanical ventilation, need to be cleaned regularly, as they are in direct contact with the patient's skin and airways. Tubing, also essential to the smooth operation of these devices, can accumulate secretions and micro-organisms, requiring special attention.

- **Daily cleaning**: The mask should be cleaned **daily** with lukewarm water and mild soap, then rinsed thoroughly and left to air dry. This step removes secretions, oils and bacteria accumulated on the mask during use.

- **Regular disinfection**: In addition to daily cleaning, weekly disinfection with specific disinfectants (alcohol-free to avoid damaging materials) is recommended to eliminate more resistant pathogens.
- **Tubing**: Tubing should be rinsed with lukewarm water and left to dry. It is essential to ensure that no moisture remains inside, as this encourages bacterial proliferation. Tubing should be **replaced** regularly, in accordance with the manufacturer's recommendations and the protocols of the healthcare facility.

## Filters and humidifiers

**Filters** and **humidifiers** are also critical elements in the management of respiratory devices. Filters, found in ventilators and CPAP/BiPAP machines, purify the air before it enters the patient's airways. If not properly maintained, they become reservoirs for dust, allergens and pathogens.

- **Filters**: CPAP/BiPAP ventilator and machine filters should be inspected regularly and changed according to the manufacturer's recommendations. Periodic cleaning is often necessary, especially for reusable filters. Single-use filters should be **replaced** regularly to avoid contaminant build-up.

- **Humidifiers**: Oxygen or ventilation humidifiers add moisture to the air to prevent mucous membranes from drying out, but they are also high-risk areas for microbial contamination if the water is not changed regularly. The water used in these tanks must be **sterile** or boiled, and the tank must be emptied and cleaned daily to prevent the growth of bacteria or fungi.

**Nebulizers**

**Nebulizers**, used to administer aerosolized drugs, must be cleaned after each use to avoid contamination by drug residues and pathogens.

- **Disassembly and cleaning**: After each nebulization session, it is essential to disassemble the device and clean each part (mouthpiece, mask, medication reservoir) with lukewarm water and mild soap, then rinse thoroughly.
- **Disinfection**: Weekly disinfection of nebulizer parts with an antiseptic solution is required. Some parts can also be sterilized by heat or steam, following the manufacturer's instructions.

## Hygiene precautions in hospitals

In hospital environments, hygiene protocols for respiratory devices must be even stricter to avoid nosocomial infections. Cross-contamination between patients is a constant risk, and specific measures are put in place to deal with it.

- **Use of single-use devices**: In high-risk departments such as intensive care, it is often recommended to use single-use devices (masks, tubing) to limit the risk of infection.

- **Inter-patient sterilization**: If reusable devices are used, they must be thoroughly disinfected or sterilized after each patient. Hospital departments follow **strict sterilization** protocols for sensitive equipment, ensuring that no pathogens remain.

- **Staff training**: Caregivers must be regularly trained in good practices for cleaning, disinfecting and managing respiratory devices. Handling errors, such as poor disinfection or forgetting to change filters, can have serious consequences for patient health.

# Patient education and prevention at home

For patients using home respiratory devices, education on hygiene practices is crucial to preventing infections. Caregivers, especially orderlies, play a key role in teaching these practices to patients and their families.

- **Cleaning instructions**: Patients should be informed of the essential steps involved in cleaning and disinfecting their equipment. This includes the use of sterile water in humidifiers, regular cleaning of masks and tubing, and the need to change filters in good time.

- **Environmental control**: It's also important to educate patients about the cleanliness of their environment. Respiratory devices should be placed in clean, well-ventilated areas. Avoiding excessive humidity, dust and smoke is essential to minimize the risk of contamination of devices and airways.

  ○ Checking connections and correct operation

**Checking that** respiratory equipment **is connected and working properly** is an essential step in the management of patients on oxygen therapy, mechanical ventilation or CPAP/BiPAP. Malfunctioning or incorrectly connected devices can have serious consequences, such as reduced oxygen supply, inadequate ventilation or air leaks, leading to a worsening of the patient's clinical condition. It is therefore essential that caregivers, and especially nursing assistants, are trained and attentive to these technical aspects, to ensure safe and effective care.

## The importance of checking connections

Respiratory devices, whether simple **nasal cannula** or **oxygen masks,** or more complex machines such as **ventilators**, CPAP and BiPAP, have a number of connections that are essential for their proper operation. These connections need to be checked regularly, as accidental disconnection, maladjustment or air leakage can compromise the correct administration of oxygen or respiratory treatment.

The purpose of checking connections is to ensure that the various components - masks, tubing, humidification tanks, filters, connections to oxygen sources or ventilation equipment - are correctly attached and working optimally.

## Checking oxygen therapy devices

For patients on **oxygen therapy**, whether fitted with nasal cannula or oxygen masks, checking oxygen connections and flow is a crucial step. Oxygen therapy is often prescribed for patients suffering from hypoxemia, and involuntary interruption of oxygen delivery can worsen dyspnea or cause complications.

### Oxygen therapy device verification steps

1. **Nasal cannula or mask connections**: It's essential to check that **nasal cannulae** are correctly positioned in the patient's nostrils, and that the tube connecting the cannula to the oxygen tank is correctly connected. Similarly, for **oxygen masks**, the mask must fit snugly around the face, perfectly covering the nose and mouth, without leaving any gaps that could lead to air leaks. Any discomfort or irritation must be adjusted immediately to ensure patient comfort.

2. **Connections to oxygen sources**: Caregivers must ensure that tubing is correctly connected to the oxygen source (cylinder, oxygen concentrator or hospital network). It is necessary to check that the connections are securely fastened, with no disconnection or leakage of oxygen, which could reduce the effectiveness of the therapy.

3. **Checking the flow meter** : The flow meter, which regulates the amount of oxygen delivered to the patient, must be checked regularly to ensure that the flow rate prescribed by the doctor is being adhered to. Accidental alteration of the flow rate could result in either insufficient oxygen (hypoxia) or excessive oxygen (hyperoxia), putting the patient at risk.

## Checking CPAP and BiPAP machines

**CPAP** (continuous positive airway pressure) and **BiPAP** (bi-level positive airway pressure) machines are used for patients suffering from sleep apnea, COPD or respiratory insufficiency. These devices maintain positive pressure in the airways to prevent collapse during sleep or improve ventilation. Correct operation of these machines depends on correct connection of the various parts and careful monitoring by the caregiver.

**CPAP/BiPAP machine verification steps**

1. **Checking the mask and tubing**: The CPAP/BiPAP mask must fit correctly over the patient's face to avoid air leaks, which could reduce the effectiveness of the treatment. It is important that the mask is neither too loose, which would result in a loss of pressure, nor too tight, which would cause discomfort or skin lesions. The **tubing** connecting the mask to the device should also be inspected to ensure that it is not twisted or obstructed.

2. **Checking the pressure setting**: The caregiver must check that the **air pressure** set on the machine corresponds to the doctor's prescription. In the case of a BiPAP, it is important to ensure that the inhalation (IPAP) and exhalation (EPAP) pressures are correctly set to optimize the patient's breathing.

3. **Air leaks and alarms**: It is essential to monitor **air leaks** around the mask, and to regularly check the machine's

alerts and alarms, which may indicate a malfunction or poor connection. Any anomaly must be corrected immediately, and the medical team informed if the problem persists.

## Checking mechanical fans

**Mechanical ventilators** are more complex devices, used for patients in intensive care or resuscitation, who require full or partial respiratory support. These machines, often connected via an endotracheal tube or tracheostomy, require constant monitoring to ensure their proper functioning.

**Checking mechanical fans**

1. **Tubing and breathing circuit connections**: The breathing circuit (including **tubing**, **filters** and **humidifiers**) must be thoroughly inspected for leaks and disconnections. Tubing must be securely attached to the ventilator and patient connections. Accidental disconnection can lead to ventilation failure, endangering the patient's life.

2. **Humidifiers and filters**: **Humidifiers**, which are used to prevent the respiratory tract from drying out, and **filters**, which purify ventilated air, must be checked regularly. Filters must be clean and securely in place, and the water in the humidifier must be sterile and changed regularly to avoid contamination.

3. **Monitoring alarms**: Mechanical ventilators are equipped with a sophisticated alarm system that signals anomalies (malfunction, poor connection, abnormal pressure, etc.). Caregivers must be trained to recognize the various alarms and respond quickly, by adjusting connections or contacting the medical team if necessary.

4. **Checking settings**: **Tidal volume**, **respiratory rate** and **air pressure** parameters should be checked regularly to ensure that the patient is receiving adequate ventilation. Any unjustified variation in parameters should be promptly reported and corrected.

## Continuous monitoring of correct operation

In addition to technical checks, **continuous monitoring of** respiratory device operation is essential. Caregivers must be alert to signs of respiratory distress in the patient (dyspnea, cyanosis, agitation), which could indicate a problem with the equipment. Likewise, it is important to carry out **regular checks** to ensure that machine settings are always adapted to the patient's condition, especially in intensive care settings where respiratory needs can change rapidly.

- **Supporting the mechanically ventilated patient**
  - Role in comfort and monitoring

The role of caregivers in the **comfort** and **monitoring** of patients using respiratory devices is fundamental. These devices, whether simple **nasal cannula** or **oxygen masks**, or more complex equipment such as **mechanical ventilators, CPAP** or **BiPAP**, can improve respiratory function, but can also generate discomfort and complications if not managed correctly. The caregiver, and in particular the nursing auxiliary, plays a crucial role in accompanying the patient, not only to ensure that treatment is effective, but also to preserve the patient's well-being and carefully monitor any changes in his or her condition.

## Role in patient comfort

**Patient comfort** with respiratory devices is essential to optimize the tolerance and efficacy of these treatments. The caregiver must therefore ensure that every aspect of the use of these devices is adapted to the patient's needs, while minimizing sources of discomfort.

**Adjusting comfort features**

- **Mask positioning**: masks used for oxygen delivery, or in CPAP and BiPAP systems, must be correctly fitted to ensure both optimum efficiency and maximum comfort. If the mask is too loose, air leaks can occur, reducing treatment efficiency. If, on the other hand, the mask is too tight, it may cause pain or skin lesions, particularly around the nose, cheeks or behind the ears. The caregiver must take care to strike a balance, adjusting the mask regularly as the patient returns.

- **Preventing skin irritation**: Areas in prolonged contact with respiratory devices, such as the nose or mouth, are particularly susceptible to **irritation** and **injury**. It's important to check the condition of the skin frequently, apply protective creams if necessary, and use protective pads or bandages to prevent rubbing. For patients on CPAP or BiPAP, who wear their mask for prolonged periods, these adjustments are particularly crucial.

- **Humidifying breathing air**: Respiratory devices can cause a sensation of dryness in the airways and mouth, particularly when dry oxygen is administered. Installing a **humidifier** on breathing circuits or oxygen therapy helps maintain adequate humidity, reducing dry mouth and nasal irritation. Caregivers should regularly check and adjust these humidification devices to ensure patient comfort.

**Patient posture and environment**

The **posture of** a patient on a respirator has a direct impact on comfort and respiratory efficiency. A patient lying uncomfortably or in the wrong position may experience respiratory discomfort, which can worsen his or her condition.

- **Semi-seated position**: The caregiver should encourage the patient to assume a **semi-seated** position, especially in patients with dyspnea or on oxygen therapy. This position, with the torso inclined at around 45 degrees, allows better thoracic expansion and relieves pressure on the diaphragm, thus facilitating breathing. This positioning is particularly recommended for patients suffering from respiratory insufficiency or COPD.

- **Quiet environment**: Respiratory comfort is also linked to the **environment**. The caregiver must ensure that the patient's environment is calm, well ventilated, and free from any source of stress or excessive noise that could aggravate dyspnea. A soothing environment promotes not only breathing, but also the patient's general well-being.

## Careful, proactive monitoring

In addition to comfort, the role of **monitoring** is fundamental to the management of respiratory devices. Careful monitoring enables early detection of any signs of aggravation or complication, guaranteeing rapid, appropriate treatment.

### Monitoring clinical signs

- **Oxygen saturation (SpO2)**: **Oxygen saturation** is one of the main indicators of the patient's proper oxygenation. The caregiver should regularly measure saturation using a pulse oximeter, ensuring that the level remains within prescribed limits (generally between 92% and 98% for patients without severe respiratory pathology). Any significant drop in SpO2 should be reported immediately to adjust oxygen flow or reassess treatment.

- **Respiratory rate**: Monitoring **respiratory rate** is essential to assess the effectiveness of the respiratory device. A respiratory rate that is too fast (tachypnea) or too slow (bradypnea) may indicate a problem, whether a worsening respiratory condition or poor device fit. The caregiver should monitor breathing continuously and report any abnormal changes.

- **Observing dyspnoea**: Visible signs of **respiratory distress** (dyspnoea, draught, use of accessory muscles) should be closely monitored. If the patient appears breathless or distressed despite the use of a respiratory device, this may indicate obstruction, worsening of the underlying disease, or equipment malfunction. In such cases, it is crucial to check the condition of the device immediately and inform the medical team.

**Device monitoring**

- **Air leaks**: Air leaks are common, especially with ventilation or oxygen therapy masks. Air leakage can reduce the effectiveness of treatment, or even render therapy totally ineffective. The caregiver should regularly check the fit of masks and tubing, ensuring that there are no leaks from fittings or valves.

- **Checking alarms**: Mechanical, CPAP and BiPAP ventilators are equipped with alarms that signal any malfunction or problem in respiratory parameters. Caregivers must be trained to recognize these alarms and intervene quickly to resolve problems, whether they be disconnections, obstructions or pressure problems.

- **Maintenance of filters and humidifiers**: Filters and humidifiers used with respiratory devices must be cleaned and changed regularly to prevent infection and ensure good quality of inspired air. Caregivers must be attentive to their condition and ensure that cleaning protocols are followed.

## Communication and psychological support

Beyond the technical aspect, the role of **psychological support** is crucial in helping patients to accept and better tolerate these sometimes intrusive devices. Patients, especially those suffering from chronic respiratory illnesses or acute respiratory failure, may feel anxious about using ventilation devices.

- **Clear, reassuring explanation**: The caregiver must provide a clear and reassuring explanation of how the device works, answering the patient's questions and allaying any fears. A good understanding of the treatment helps to reduce anxiety and encourage patient cooperation.

- **Encouraging active participation**: Encouraging patients to take an active part in their care, for example by adjusting their own masks or expressing their feelings, helps reinforce their autonomy and reduce the feeling of dependence.

  ○    Signs of discomfort and rapid intervention
**Signs of discomfort** in patients using respiratory devices such as **ventilators**, **CPAPs**, **BiPAPs** or undergoing **oxygen therapy** must be identified promptly to ensure not only patient comfort, but also treatment efficacy. A patient who is uncomfortable or in pain is less likely to tolerate these devices properly, which can compromise their management. **Prompt** intervention is essential to prevent further discomfort or more serious complications. The caregiver's role in detecting these signs and managing the situation is crucial.

## Signs of discomfort

Signs of discomfort in a patient on respiratory support may be subtle, but they should never be ignored. They may be **physical**, **behavioral** or linked to **changes in vital parameters**. Knowing and recognizing these signs is essential for rapid intervention.

### Physical signs of discomfort

- **Skin lesions and irritation**: Breathing devices such as masks or tubing can cause irritation or redness at points of contact with the skin, particularly around the nose, cheeks and behind the ears. The appearance of **sores** or **bedsores** in these areas is a sign of excessive pressure or poor mask fit. Regular monitoring of the skin around the devices is therefore essential.

- **Dry mucous membranes**: Air delivered by respiratory devices can cause **dry mouth** or nose, leading to burning, discomfort or even **lesions** in the nostrils. Mucous membrane dryness is often aggravated by prolonged use of oxygen without humidification, or by excessively high oxygen flow rates.

- **Pain**: A patient may experience **chest**, abdominal or facial **pain** due to the pressure exerted by the devices or the effort required to breathe with the device. For example, prolonged use of ventilators or CPAP may cause discomfort in the respiratory muscles.

### Behavioral signs

- **Agitation and anxiety**: Respiratory discomfort may cause **agitation**, incessant movement or attempts to remove the mask or device. This agitation is often associated with **increasing anxiety**, particularly in patients with dyspnea, as they may feel suffocated or trapped by respiratory equipment.

158

- **Refusal or intolerance of the device**: Some patients express their discomfort by refusing to wear the device, repeatedly trying to remove it, or verbally expressing their discomfort. This is particularly common in patients on CPAP or BiPAP, where the sensation of continuous air pressure can be perceived as intrusive or unpleasant.

**Changes in vital parameters**

- **Abnormal respiratory rate**: A patient in discomfort may show an **increase in respiratory rate** (tachypnea) due to respiratory discomfort. Conversely, some may breathe more slowly or superficially, in an attempt to minimize discomfort.

- **Changes in oxygen saturation**: A drop in **oxygen saturation (SpO2)** may occur due to poor tolerance to the device, air leakage or malfunction. If the patient is uncomfortable, the effectiveness of the therapy may be compromised, leading to a drop in SpO2.

# Quick response

Once signs of discomfort have been identified, rapid intervention is crucial to resolving the situation and ensuring the patient's well-being. A **rapid response** not only restores the patient's comfort, but also prevents a worsening of their clinical condition or a reduction in the effectiveness of treatment.

**Device adjustment**

- **Mask readjustment**: If the mask or tubing is incorrectly positioned, leading to painful pressure points or air leaks, the first reflex is to **readjust the equipment**. The caregiver should check that the mask fits snugly, without being too tight, and that it does not exert excessive pressure on the skin. If irritation or skin lesions are present, it may be necessary to change the type of mask or add **protection** such as pads.

- **Humidifying the air**: In the event of dry mouth or nose, adding or adjusting a **humidifier** to the respiratory system can help alleviate symptoms. If a humidifier is already in place, the caregiver should check that it is working properly and that the sterile water level is sufficient. This simple modification often greatly improves patient comfort.

- **Adjusting air flow or pressure**: In the case of CPAP, BiPAP or ventilator devices, it may be necessary to adjust **air pressure** or oxygen flow if the patient complains of respiratory discomfort or shows signs of insufficient tolerance. This must be done under the supervision of the medical team, as incorrect adjustment can compromise the effectiveness of respiratory therapy.

**Application of comfort care**

- **Mucous membrane hydration**: For patients with dry mouth or nose, **moisturizing sprays** or **saline solutions** can be applied to relieve irritated mucous membranes. It is also important to maintain good general hydration by encouraging the patient to drink small amounts of water regularly.

- **Skin care**: If skin irritation occurs around areas of contact with the device, applying **moisturizing creams** or **protective ointments** can prevent further damage and soothe the skin. If wounds are present, it is important to apply suitable dressings and readjust the device to limit friction.

**Psychological support and reassurance**

The discomfort felt by patients on respiratory devices is often exacerbated by **anxiety** linked to their respiratory situation. The role of the caregiver is therefore not limited to technical adjustment of the equipment, but includes genuine **psychological support**.

- **Reassuring communication**: It's important to reassure the patient by clearly explaining the steps involved in the procedure, and offering explanations of how the device works. Clear, benevolent communication helps to allay anxieties linked to the sensation of lack of air or the presence of the device on the face.

- **Encouraging cooperation**: If the patient is agitated or refuses to wear the device, it's crucial to gently encourage him/her to cooperate, explaining that these adjustments are being made to improve comfort and safety. The caregiver can also suggest pauses if possible, so that the patient can catch his or her breath before readjusting the device.

## Monitoring and reassessment

After the procedure, it is essential to **closely monitor** the patient's condition to ensure that the adjustments made have indeed improved comfort and clinical status. It is also necessary to check whether signs of discomfort or respiratory distress persist.

- **Reassess vital signs**: Once adjustments have been made, the caregiver should recheck **vital signs** (oxygen saturation, respiratory rate, heart rate) to ensure that the device is correctly calibrated and that the patient is receiving adequate oxygen.

- **Ongoing monitoring**: Regular monitoring of the patient is necessary to detect any new signs of discomfort. The patient should also be encouraged to report any discomfort or pain as soon as it occurs, so that adjustments can be made in a timely manner.

# Chapter 7

# Supporting patients with chronic illnesses

- **Living with chronic respiratory disease**
  - ○ Psychological and social impact of chronic diseases

**Chronic diseases** have a profound impact not only on the physical, but also on the **psychological** and **social** dimensions of patients' lives. Living with a long-term condition, whether it's a respiratory disease such as **COPD**, **diabetes**, or cardiovascular disease, affects the way individuals perceive themselves, interact with others, and envisage their future. These diseases are more than just physiological symptoms; they profoundly alter quality of life, and can have significant psychological and social consequences.

# The psychological impact of chronic illness

The diagnosis and long-term management of a chronic illness are often accompanied by an **emotional shock** and a series of psychological adjustments. The impact may vary according to the individual, the severity of the illness, and the support available, but certain psychological elements are frequently found in people with chronic illnesses.

## Anxiety and depression

**Anxiety** and **depressive disorders** are frequent psychological consequences of chronic illness. The feeling of losing control over one's body and health, uncertainty about the course of the disease and fear of complications can generate constant **anxiety**. Patients often feel overwhelmed by the day-to-day management of their disease: regular medication, frequent medical follow-up, and necessary lifestyle adjustments. This can create chronic stress, sometimes difficult to manage.

Depression can also set in for people with chronic illnesses, particularly when the disease significantly impairs their ability to lead an active, independent life. Feelings of helplessness, isolation and being a burden to others contribute to this depressive picture. In some patients, depression may also be exacerbated by

164

physical symptoms, such as chronic fatigue or pain, which limit activities and create a negative spiral.

**Loss of self-esteem and identity**

Living with a chronic illness can profoundly alter a person's sense of self. Patients may experience a **loss of identity**, particularly if the disease affects their ability to work, socialize or participate in activities that were once an integral part of their lives. For example, a previously active person who now suffers from breathing difficulties due to a disease like COPD may feel diminished, frustrated, even useless.

This loss of self-esteem is often linked to an inability to meet personal or societal expectations. Patients may find it difficult to accept their physical limitations and redefine their place in society, leading to feelings of shame or failure. Self-perception changes, from a person in full possession of his or her means to one perceived as fragile or dependent.

**Fear of the future**

**Uncertainty about the course of the disease** is a major source of psychological stress. Patients often wonder how their disease will progress, what the next steps will be, and how their quality of life will deteriorate over time. This fear of the future is accompanied by worries about loss of autonomy and the growing need for assistance. It can also include anxieties about access to care, the costs associated with the disease, or the possibility of becoming a burden to loved ones.

# Social impact of chronic diseases

Chronic illnesses not only affect the individual sphere, they also change **social relationships**, participation in community life and the role patients play in their family, work and social circle.

**Social isolation**

One of the most striking effects of chronic illness is **social isolation**. Patients, especially those with respiratory illnesses or chronic pain, may be forced to limit their outings and interactions because of their physical condition. Symptoms such as fatigue, dyspnea or pain make social activities trying. Patients may refuse to go out, attend social events or meet friends, not because they lack interest, but because their illness physically prevents them from doing so.

This social isolation is often reinforced by a feeling of embarrassment or shame, especially when the disease is visible or perceived as stigmatizing. Some patients are afraid of being pitied or judged by those around them because of their physical limitations, leading them to isolate themselves even further. This situation can create a **rupture with the social network**, fuelling feelings of loneliness and exacerbating psychological disorders such as depression.

**Changes in family relationships**

Chronic illnesses also transform **family dynamics**. A patient who was once the breadwinner of his or her family may find themselves dependent on loved ones for activities of daily living, such as grooming, medication management or transportation. This can generate **discomfort** and **feelings of guilt** in patients, who feel they are losing their role as protector or provider, and becoming a burden to their loved ones.

On the other hand, the family can also come under **increased pressure**. Family members often become **caregivers**, a heavy responsibility that can lead to stress, exhaustion and relationship conflicts. Relatives have to reorganize their lives to include caring for the sick person, which can have repercussions on their own activities and relationships. Thus, chronic illness affects not only the patient, but also the whole of his or her entourage.

## Impact on professional life

Patients suffering from chronic illnesses can experience significant **difficulties at work**. The inability to maintain a regular work rhythm, due to symptoms or frequent medical appointments, can lead to a **reduction in working hours**, or even a total inability to continue their professional activity. This can lead to **financial loss**, a feeling of worthlessness, and a weakening of self-esteem, especially if work used to be part of the patient's social and personal identity.

In some cases, the **stigma** attached to chronic illness can also play a role in marginalizing patients in the workplace. Colleagues or employers may, even unintentionally, treat a chronically ill person differently, reinforcing isolation or feelings of inadequacy. This can lead some patients to choose to hide their illness, at the risk of worsening their condition.

## Coping and support strategies

To cope with the psychological and social impacts of chronic illness, **coping strategies** and **support systems** are essential.

- **Psychological support**: Psychological support, whether in the form of individual therapy, support groups or psychiatric follow-up, can be a great help to patients. Managing the emotions associated with the disease, such as anxiety and depression, helps patients to come to terms with the situation and regain a better quality of life.

- **Family and social** support: Maintaining an **active social network** is crucial to avoid isolation. Encouraging participation in support groups or patient associations helps to exchange experiences and break the solitude. Family support is also central, and it is important for relatives to be informed about the disease so that they can offer appropriate support without becoming emotionally overburdened.

- **Lifestyle adaptation**: Adjustments to daily routine, including adapted physical activity, stress management strategies, and better organization of medical care, can help maintain a balance between disease management and participation in pleasurable activities.

  ◦ The importance of continuous, empathetic care

The **importance of continuous, empathic care** for patients suffering from illnesses, whether acute or chronic, cannot be overstated. An approach that combines **regular medical follow-up** with **empathy** not only ensures effective medical treatment, but also supports the patient's psychological and emotional well-being. This creates a care environment in which the patient feels **listened to**, **understood** and **supported**, thus promoting better adherence to treatment and improved quality of life.

## Continuity of care: a key to therapeutic effectiveness

**Continuity of care** is essential, especially for patients with chronic or progressive illnesses. Unlike ad hoc care, continuity enables **regular monitoring** of disease progression, treatment responses and the adjustments needed to optimize therapeutic outcomes. This close, regular monitoring is crucial to preventing complications, detecting warning signals early and adapting treatments proactively.

### Preventing complications

When care is provided on an ongoing basis, caregivers are able to detect **complications** or signs of worsening disease at an early stage. For example, in a **COPD** patient, a sudden exacerbation of symptoms, such as an increase in dyspnea or a drop in oxygen saturation, can be identified and treated early, thus avoiding hospitalization. Similarly, in patients with **diabetes**, regular monitoring can help manage blood sugar levels more effectively, and prevent serious complications such as neuropathy or kidney failure.

Continuous care is based on personalized monitoring of **vital signs**, general clinical condition and any side effects of treatment. This vigilance, combined with rapid, appropriate adjustments, optimizes management and ensures a better quality of life for the patient.

**Improved treatment compliance**

Ongoing management also plays a crucial role in **treatment adherence**. For many patients, managing a chronic disease involves complex treatments, lifestyle changes, or a strict medication routine. Without support and follow-up, it can be difficult for patients to scrupulously adhere to these requirements. On the other hand, regular care, in which the caregiver takes the time to check that treatments are being properly understood and applied, helps to **reinforce the** patient's **commitment** to his or her own care.

Regular dialogue with the caregiver, individualized adjustments and the reassurance that progress is being monitored and recognized all contribute to strengthening the patient's confidence in the treatment and improving **therapeutic compliance**. They feel less alone in the face of their illness, and more encouraged to continue their efforts.

## Empathy: a fundamental element of care

**Empathy** is at the heart of any quality healthcare relationship. It creates a **bond of trust** between patient and caregiver, a bond that goes beyond medical treatments and diagnoses to encompass consideration of the patient's **emotions**, **worries** and **fears**. This holistic approach is crucial to the patient's well-being, and contributes directly to effective care.

## Understanding the patient experience

Every patient's experience of illness is unique. For some, chronic illness is a constant source of anxiety; for others, it may be experienced as an attack on their identity or a loss of autonomy. Empathy enables caregivers to place themselves in the patient's perspective, to understand his or her fears, limitations and expectations. It's about seeing the patient as a whole, not just through his or her illness.

For example, a **cancer** patient may feel immense anxiety about the uncertainty of his or her future, or fear the side effects of heavy treatments such as chemotherapy. Empathy enables the caregiver to recognize these concerns and adapt their approach to offer emotional support in addition to medical treatment. This can include regular conversations about the patient's emotional state, space to express fears, and gestures of comfort that go beyond the simple administration of medication.

## Active listening and benevolent communication

Empathetic care is based on **active listening** and **benevolent communication**. Active listening involves not only paying attention to the patient's words, but also picking up on **non-verbal signs** of distress or discomfort, such as agitation, fatigue or frustration. Empathy prompts the caregiver to ask open-ended questions to understand the patient's feelings, and to respond with compassion and patience to his or her concerns.

**Good communication** helps to establish a climate of trust and security. It involves speaking to the patient in a respectful manner, avoiding incomprehensible medical jargon, and clearly explaining each stage of the treatment or examination. This reassures patients and helps them better understand their illness and what is being done to manage it.

**Emotional support**

Empathetic care includes ongoing **emotional support**. Patients with chronic or serious illnesses often experience emotional ups and downs. By being present and offering emotional support, the caregiver enables the patient to overcome difficult moments, such as relapses or periods of uncertainty. This can take the form of words of encouragement, validation of the patient's feelings, or simply an attentive presence.

This emotional support has a direct impact on how patients cope with their illness. It has been shown that patients who feel emotionally supported are better able to manage disease-related stress, tolerate treatment better and have a more positive outlook on their future.

# The link between continuity, empathy and quality of life

The combination of **continuous care** and an **empathetic approach** creates a framework in which the patient feels cared for as a whole, on both a medical and a human level. This approach improves not only the patient's physical condition, but also his or her **quality of life**.

### Improved quality of life

Ongoing care **stabilizes** the patient's condition, reduces the frequency of exacerbations or complications, and provides ongoing support in managing daily symptoms. In turn, empathy and benevolent communication improve the patient's psychological and emotional well-being, reducing the stress and anxiety associated with the disease. This promotes greater resilience in the face of daily challenges, whether pain, fatigue or managing the stresses of treatment.

For example, a patient with long-term **diabetes**, regularly monitored and supported by empathetic caregivers, will be more likely to manage his or her diet and insulin treatment well and remain motivated in his or her management, thus improving overall quality of life.

**Strengthening the patient-caregiver relationship**

The bond of trust between patient and caregiver is strengthened when an empathetic approach is adopted. This bond is essential if the patient is to feel safe and understood. By feeling supported, the patient is more inclined to share his or her difficulties or express doubts, enabling the caregiver to provide more appropriate solutions and make the necessary adjustments. This relationship also strengthens the patient's commitment to his or her own health, by creating a partnership in which the caregiver accompanies and supports the patient in managing his or her illness.

- **Patient and family education**
  - Encourage autonomy: use of home oxygen, breathing techniques

**Encouraging autonomy** in patients with chronic respiratory diseases, who require the use of home oxygen and the learning of specific breathing techniques, is a fundamental approach to improving their quality of life. The aim is to enable patients to regain a degree of control over their health, actively participate in the management of their disease and minimize their dependence on carers or relatives. By helping patients to master **home oxygen therapy** and practice appropriate **breathing techniques**, we promote their **autonomy, self-confidence** and **daily well-being**.

# Home oxygen therapy: autonomous management

For patients suffering from respiratory diseases such as **COPD**, **emphysema** or other lung-limiting conditions, **home oxygen therapy** is often an integral part of their treatment. The use of portable oxygen concentrators or cylinders helps maintain adequate blood oxygen levels, essential for organ health and quality of life. Autonomy in managing this therapy is crucial to enable patients to lead as normal a life as possible.

## Teaching the use of devices

One of the first steps in encouraging autonomy is to ensure that the patient understands how to use oxygen therapy devices correctly. This includes clear explanations of **installation**, **maintenance** and **operation** of concentrators or portable oxygen cylinders.

- **Assembly and adjustment**: Patients need to be trained to **assemble** and **disassemble** their **device**, to connect tubing and masks correctly, and to adjust the **oxygen flow** themselves according to medical prescriptions. This mastery enables patients to manage their treatment with confidence, without the need for constant third-party intervention.

- **Monitoring oxygen levels**: It's also crucial to teach patients how to monitor **oxygen saturation** using a pulse oximeter, to check that levels remain within recommended values. This enables them to quickly detect any drop in saturation and react by adjusting their oxygen intake or contacting a healthcare professional if necessary.

- **Device maintenance**: Device maintenance, such as cleaning filters, refilling humidifiers and replacing worn parts, is also part of the skills to be taught. With autonomy over maintenance, patients are less dependent on external assistance and can maintain effective treatment on a daily basis.

**Manage oxygen therapy independently**

Once the basics of oxygen therapy have been mastered, the next step is to **integrate the use of oxygen** into the patient's daily routine, so as to reduce the discomfort and potential isolation it can cause.

- **Mobility with oxygen**: Oxygen therapy at home should not be a barrier to mobility or social activities. By using portable devices )lightweight oxygen cylinders or mobile concentrators), patients can continue to move around outdoors, take part in social activities and get out of the house. Encouraging patients to use oxygen in a variety of contexts, both at home and outdoors, is essential to help them maintain their independence.

- **Planning and anticipation**: Another important aspect of autonomy is the ability to **plan oxygen use** according to planned activities. This includes managing oxygen levels according to the effort involved (e.g., increasing flow slightly when walking), planning travel with spare cylinders or portable concentrators, and managing unforeseen situations.

## Learning breathing techniques: a tool for autonomy

In parallel with oxygen therapy, learning adapted **breathing techniques** enables patients to better manage their dyspnea, reduce their anxiety about breathlessness and maximize the efficiency of their respiratory function. These techniques offer a non-pharmacological means of improving respiratory capacity and promoting autonomy in symptom management.

## Controlled breathing techniques

**Controlled breathing techniques** are particularly effective for patients suffering from chronic respiratory diseases. These methods help reduce breathlessness and regulate breathing during daily activities.

- **Pursed-lip breathing**: This technique consists of inhaling slowly through the nose, then exhaling gently through the mouth, pursing the lips as if blowing through a straw. This helps to keep the **airways open** longer, eliminate stale air more efficiently and improve gas exchange. This technique is often used during attacks of dyspnea, enabling patients to regain control of their breathing in stressful situations.

- **Diaphragmatic breathing**: **Diaphragmatic**, or abdominal, breathing involves using the diaphragm rather than the intercostal muscles. This makes for deeper, more efficient breathing. Patients place their hands on their abdomen to feel the movement of air, and concentrate on slow, deep breaths. This technique improves lung capacity and reduces the sensation of breathlessness.

These methods need to be practised regularly, so that the patient can integrate them naturally into his or her daily life, especially during times of effort or stress.

## Exercise training and dyspnea management

**Exercise retraining** is another key component of respiratory autonomy. Patients with chronic diseases can quickly lose confidence in their ability to perform physical activities due to dyspnea. By relearning how to manage their breathing during exercise, they can regain a more satisfactory level of activity.

- **Effort planning**: Using controlled breathing techniques, patients can be encouraged to plan their efforts and split up activities that require more energy (e.g. climbing stairs slowly, taking regular breaks). This approach makes it possible to manage fatigue while remaining active.

- **Managing breathlessness-related panic**: For many patients, breathlessness is a source of anxiety. Mastering controlled breathing techniques, combined with awareness of the warning signs of dyspnoea, helps to manage moments of breathlessness more effectively. Patients learn **to anticipate and react** to dyspnea rather than panic, improving their self-confidence and ability to stay active.

## Psychological and social benefits of autonomy

Encouraging autonomy in the use of home oxygen and the practice of breathing techniques has a considerable impact on patients' **psychological well-being** and **social life**.

### Boosting self-confidence

A sense of **control** over one's illness is a key factor in boosting **self-confidence**. When a patient masters the use of oxygen, knows how to manage his symptoms and can adapt his efforts without fear of breathlessness, he regains some of his independence. This improves self-esteem and reduces anxiety linked to the disease.

### Reducing dependency

By being able to independently manage their oxygen therapy and breathing techniques, patients are less dependent on those around them for daily activities. This reduction in dependence is a key factor in restoring a satisfactory **quality of life**, particularly for patients who wish to remain active and independent in their own homes.

**Maintaining social relations**

Autonomy in disease management also enables patients to **maintain social interactions**. The ability to leave home with a portable oxygen device, to participate in activities without fear of dyspnea, or to better control respiratory symptoms during conversations and social gatherings reduces isolation. This enables the patient to maintain family and friendships, which are essential for good mental health.

      ◦   Emotional support and practical advice

**Emotional support** and **practical advice** play a fundamental role in the management of patients with chronic or serious illnesses. Although the medical aspect is central to treatment, it is not enough on its own to enable patients to fully manage their illness. Particular attention must be paid to the **emotional dimension** of care, as illness impacts not only the body, but also the mind, social relationships and quality of life. Offering emotional support and appropriate practical advice enables us to accompany patients in a more holistic way, taking into account their psychological needs, fears and doubts.

## The importance of emotional support

When a person is faced with a chronic illness, whether respiratory, cardiac or metabolic, the emotional impact can be as profound as the physical symptoms. Fear of the disease's progression, the limitations imposed by it and uncertainty about the future can lead to feelings of **stress**, **anxiety** and even **depression**. It is therefore crucial to provide emotional support to these patients to help them navigate these feelings and accompany them on their journey.

### Active listening and empathy

The first pillar of emotional support is **active listening**. This means being fully attentive to the patient's words and feelings, without judging or rushing. Active listening involves asking open-ended questions, giving the patient the space to express his or her emotions, and responding with empathy.

- **Make yourself available**: An attentive, caring presence helps patients to feel **heard** and **understood**, which is fundamental to building a relationship of trust. For example, a COPD patient may express feelings of frustration at his loss of mobility, or a sense of fear linked to constant breathlessness. Enabling them to verbalize these feelings without minimizing them is essential to providing effective emotional support.

- **Validating emotions**: It's important to **validate** the patient's emotions by acknowledging the difficulty of the situation. Saying phrases like "I understand how difficult this is for you" or "it's normal to feel this way" can go a long way towards legitimizing what the patient is experiencing. This shows the patient that they are not alone in their suffering, and that their feelings are understandable and shared by others in similar situations.

**Encouraging emotional expression**

Many patients with chronic illnesses may find it difficult to express their **emotions**, especially if they are negative. Some may fear becoming a "burden" to those around them, or feel uncomfortable expressing fear or sadness. Encouraging patients to share their emotions can relieve some of the psychological burden they may be carrying.

- **Creating a climate of safety**: It's essential to create a space where the patient feels **safe** to talk. This can include regular moments of discussion about the patient's emotional state, without necessarily focusing on the medical aspect. This helps to identify signs of anxiety or depression that may require further support.

178

- **Facilitating family support**: In addition to the support provided by caregivers, it is important to help patients **involve their loved ones** in this emotional dimension. Encouraging open communication within the family or social circle helps patients to avoid feeling isolated by their illness. Relatives can also play a key role in providing emotional support and helping to lighten the patient's emotional load.

## Practical advice for day-to-day disease management

In addition to emotional support, patients often need **practical advice** on how to manage their disease on a day-to-day basis. Such advice helps patients to maintain a certain degree of autonomy and to better adapt to the challenges posed by their condition. Offering concrete recommendations adapted to everyday life can make managing the disease less overwhelming.

### Structuring your daily routine

One of the main challenges of chronic illness is adapting one's life to a new physical reality. Structuring an adapted daily routine helps to manage symptoms more effectively, while minimizing the impact of the disease on everyday life.

- **Planning activities**: It is often necessary for patients to organize their days around their illness. For example, for a patient suffering from dyspnea, it can be useful to plan **rest periods** after strenuous activities, such as climbing stairs or moving around. Learning to divide up efforts and avoid stressful situations helps to better manage symptoms, while enabling patients to remain active.

- **Fatigue management**: Chronic illness is often accompanied by significant fatigue. Practical advice on fatigue management can include arranging **short naps**, prioritizing essential activities, and using tools or technical

179

aids to reduce physical load, such as wheelchairs for long distances or household appliances to facilitate daily tasks.

## Advice on treatment management

Drug treatments and other therapies associated with chronic disease management can be complex. Offering practical advice on how to organize and follow treatment can help reduce errors and improve **compliance**.

- **Use of reminders**: For patients taking multiple medications or undergoing specific treatments, **reminders** (alarms on the phone, compartmentalized medication boxes) can help ensure that they don't forget to take their medication on time. This can also include advice on how to manage side effects, or information on the possible interaction between medication and diet.

- **Monitoring vital parameters**: For patients needing to monitor vital constants, such as **oxygen saturation** or **blood pressure**, practical advice on how to use devices (oximeters, blood pressure monitors) and how to keep a diary of results can promote rigorous, autonomous monitoring. This enables patients to play an active role in their own disease management.

## Adapting the living environment

The daily environment of a patient suffering from a chronic disease often needs to be adapted to facilitate symptom management and prevent the risk of complications.

- **Home reorganization**: It is often **advisable** to **reorganize the living space** to facilitate movement and limit the risk of falls or fatigue. For example, for a patient suffering from respiratory problems, installing grab bars in the bathroom, or using seats in the shower, can make everyday movements easier and safer. Similarly, reducing obstacles in the home can help limit unnecessary effort.

- **Consideration of nutritional needs**: Patients with chronic diseases can benefit from specific nutritional advice. In some cases, it may be necessary to **modify the diet** to better meet energy requirements, reduce weight gain or prevent complications. An adapted food plan can be drawn up to ensure that patients have the energy they need to manage their disease, while avoiding excesses or deficiencies.

# Impact of emotional support and practical advice on quality of life

Constant **emotional support**, combined with appropriate **practical advice**, significantly improves the **quality of life of** patients with chronic illnesses. By helping patients to manage not only the medical aspects, but also the emotional and practical challenges of their illness, they can feel more autonomous, more in control of their condition, and better equipped to cope with everyday difficulties.

### Empowerment

Emotional support and practical advice help **empower** patients. By giving them the tools to manage their own treatment and lifestyle, patients regain a sense of control over their lives, despite their illness. This autonomy, whether in managing symptoms, treatments or the environment, enables them to maintain an active and dignified life, while limiting their dependence on others.

### Reduced stress and anxiety

Knowing that you have the practical and emotional means to cope with your illness significantly reduces **stress** and **anxiety**. When patients feel supported and well advised, they are less likely to panic in the event of unexpected symptoms or complications. This confidence in their ability to manage their disease has a positive effect on their mental and physical well-being.

- **End-of-life care for respiratory diseases**
  - Palliative care in pneumology

**Palliative care in pulmonology** plays a fundamental role in the management of patients with advanced and incurable respiratory diseases, such as **COPD, pulmonary fibrosis** and **bronchial cancer**. The aim of palliative care is not to cure the disease, but to relieve symptoms, improve quality of life and offer emotional, psychological and spiritual support to patients and their families. In respirology, where chronic respiratory illness often leads to significant respiratory distress and a major impact on daily life, palliative care helps patients to manage pain, shortness of breath and other disabling symptoms, while ensuring a humane and empathetic approach to the end of life.

## Relieving physical symptoms

Advanced respiratory diseases cause severe symptoms, including **shortness of breath (dyspnea), pain, fatigue,** and sometimes **persistent coughing** or copious **bronchial secretions**. These symptoms can be very disabling, limiting the patient's mobility and affecting his or her ability to lead as normal a life as possible. The aim of palliative care is to reduce these symptoms and offer the patient **optimum comfort**.

## Dyspnea management

**Shortness of breath** is one of the most distressing symptoms for patients with advanced lung disease. Even at rest, patients suffering from **severe COPD** or **pulmonary fibrosis** can experience severe dyspnea, generating a feeling of suffocation that increases anxiety and stress.

- **Oxygen therapy**: One of the main interventions to relieve dyspnea is **oxygen therapy**. In patients with end-stage respiratory failure, oxygen administered at home or in hospital helps maintain sufficient oxygen saturation, which in turn helps reduce breathlessness. This is accompanied by regular monitoring and adjustment of the oxygen flow according to the evolution of symptoms.

- **Medications**: Respiratory palliative care also uses **medications** to relieve dyspnea, including low-dose **opioids** such as morphine, which, in addition to reducing pain, helps reduce the sensation of breathlessness by altering the brain's perception of oxygen deprivation. Benzodiazepines **can** be prescribed to calm anxiety linked to dyspnea.

- **Breathing techniques: Controlled breathing techniques**, such as pursed-lip breathing, are taught to help patients better control their breathing and reduce shortness of breath during attacks. This improves effort tolerance and reduces anxiety linked to the sensation of suffocation.

## Pain management

In patients with **bronchial cancer** or lung disease with complications, pain is another frequent symptom. **Palliative care** aims to provide adequate management of this pain, so that the patient can maintain a certain quality of life.

- **Analgesics**: Pain is often treated with **analgesics** adapted to the intensity of symptoms, ranging from mild analgesics such as paracetamol to more powerful **opioids** in cases of intense pain. These treatments are regularly adjusted to maintain good pain control while minimizing side effects.

- **Non-medicinal care**: **Non-medicinal approaches** such as massage, gentle physiotherapy or heat application can also help relieve certain types of pain, particularly in patients suffering from muscle tension associated with difficult breathing.

**Managing bronchial secretions**

Patients suffering from terminal respiratory illnesses can experience an **accumulation of bronchial secretions**, making breathing even more difficult and causing exhausting coughing fits.

- **Bronchial suctioning**: For some patients, **bronchial suctioning** may be necessary to clear the airways and improve respiratory comfort. Aspiration must be performed with care to avoid additional discomfort.

- **Mucolytics and humidification**: **Mucolytics** can be administered to thin secretions and facilitate their evacuation. The use of a **humidifier** may also be recommended to prevent mucous membranes from drying out and reduce mucus accumulation.

## Emotional and spiritual support

Chronic respiratory illnesses, especially in the terminal phase, can cause considerable **psychological** and **spiritual suffering**, both for the patient and his or her loved ones. Fear of breathlessness, progressive loss of autonomy and the prospect of death are all sources of **anxiety**, **depression** and even **despair**. Palliative care is not just about alleviating physical symptoms, but also providing in-depth support to help patients live through this period with **dignity** and **serenity**.

## Psychological support

Psychological support in palliative care in pneumology is essential. Patients must be able to express their fears, doubts and **confusion** about the disease and the end of life.

- **Listening and communication**: Caregivers must offer **attentive**, caring **listening**, encouraging patients to verbalize their emotions and concerns. Creating a space where patients feel safe to talk about their suffering can help reduce emotional isolation and make the last moments of life more comfortable.

- **Support for the family**: Support also concerns the patient's **family**, who often experience great distress when faced with the deteriorating state of their loved one's health. Caregivers play a key role in explaining the progression of the disease, offering psychological support and facilitating communication within the family to anticipate the decisions to be made.

## Spiritual support

Beyond the psychological aspect, patients in the palliative phase sometimes feel the need to find **meaning** in their experience, or to **reconnect with their spiritual** or religious **values**. Palliative care offers a framework for meeting these spiritual needs, whether religious or more personal.

- **Respect for beliefs**: It is essential that the palliative care team respects the patient's **beliefs** and **values**, whatever they may be, and facilitates access to spiritual support if the patient feels the need. This may include the presence of religious leaders, the organization of rituals or simply the opportunity for the patient to reflect on his or her own beliefs and the meaning of life.

# Preparing for the end of life and supporting loved ones

One of the central missions of **palliative care** in pulmonology is to prepare patients and their families for the **end of life**. The prospect of death is often a difficult subject to broach, but in palliative care it's crucial to do so with **sensitivity** and **respect**, in order to ease anxieties as much as possible.

### Preparing the patient

Preparing for the end of life does not mean abandoning the patient, but rather accompanying them in their final moments with kindness and care. The emphasis is on **respecting the** patient's **wishes** and creating a care environment that respects his or her needs and wishes.

- **Advance directives**: One important aspect is to help patients formulate **advance directives**, clearly expressing their wishes in terms of treatment (or cessation of treatment) as their illness progresses. This ensures that the patient's autonomy is respected right to the end, and relieves those close to him/her of the burden of difficult decisions.

### Supporting loved ones

The patient's loved ones play a crucial role, but they themselves can be overwhelmed by suffering and the imminence of loss. Palliative care in pulmonology provides **specific support** for families, enabling them to find support, be informed about the stages ahead and be prepared for the loss.

- **Psychological support**: Palliative care teams provide **psychological support** to families, helping them to get through this period of accompaniment with greater serenity. This includes regular discussion sessions, meetings with psychologists, and the creation of rest areas for relatives in care centers.

○    The caregiver's key role in supporting families
**Caregivers** play a fundamental role in **supporting families** throughout a patient's course of care, particularly when the patient is suffering from a serious illness or is in the palliative phase. The caregiver's presence is often an essential support for families at times of great uncertainty, anxiety and even distress. As a privileged member of the care team, the caregiver acts as a **direct contact**, a **point of reference** and a **source of comfort** for families, while facilitating communication between loved ones, the patient and the medical team. Their role is not limited to caring for the patient: they also provide psychological and practical support to the family, helping them to better understand the medical situation, manage their emotions and participate in the care process.

## A privileged point of contact

In hospital or home care, the caregiver is often the person who is most present with the patient and his or her family on a day-to-day basis. He or she is the first to **answer** relatives' **questions**, **listen to their concerns** and provide a space where they can express their feelings. This proximity to the family makes the caregiver a **privileged point of contact**, acting as a **mediator** between the family and the rest of the care team.

### Providing accessible information

Families can feel lost or overwhelmed by the complexity of medical care. The caregiver is there to **provide clear, accessible information**, explaining in simple terms what is happening with the patient. For example, when the family doesn't understand changes in the patient's condition or new medical interventions, the caregiver can describe in understandable terms what has been decided and why.

- **Explanation of care**: If a treatment is introduced, such as oxygen or infusions, the caregiver can explain to the family how it works and what it is intended to achieve. This helps to **allay concerns** about the appearance of medical equipment or the perceived worsening of the patient's condition.

- **Clarity on symptoms**: When the patient presents worrying symptoms, such as shortness of breath or pain, the caregiver can reassure the family that these signs are being managed and that specific measures are being implemented to relieve the patient.

**Building trust**

**Trust** is a key element in the relationship between caregiver and family. Families, often anxious and in search of answers, naturally turn to the caregiver who, thanks to his or her regular presence, becomes a trusted figure. This relationship is built **on active listening**, caring and professionalism.

- **Listening to concerns**: The caregiver's availability enables families to express their fears and doubts. Whether these are fears linked to the patient's suffering, the progression of the disease or the end of life, the caregiver is there to **listen without judgment** and provide comfort. This creates a strong emotional bond, enabling families to feel supported at this difficult time.

- **Assurance and reassurance**: When the family is prey to anxiety, the caregiver plays a reassuring role, reminding them that the patient is well cared for, that every intervention is carried out for their comfort, and that the medical team remains attentive to the evolution of their condition. This **reassuring presence** helps to ease tension and provide a form of emotional security for the family.

# Offer emotional support

Families faced with the serious illness or end of life of a loved one experience moments of intense emotion. They may go through different emotional phases, such as **shock**, **denial**, **anger**, **sadness**, **resignation** or **acceptance**. The caregiver, by virtue of his or her daily proximity to the family, is often the **privileged witness of** these emotions, and has a key role to play in providing **psychological support**.

### Welcoming emotions

The caregiver must be able to **recognize and welcome the emotions** of loved ones, without seeking to minimize or ignore them. When dealing with families in distress, it is essential to **legitimize their feelings** and allow them to express them freely.

- **Welcoming sadness**: When a patient is terminally ill, families may feel great sadness at the prospect of loss. The caregiver can offer them a **compassionate listening** space, allowing them to share their pain while supporting them with **empathy** and **kindness**.

- **Dealing with anger or frustration**: Some families, faced with powerlessness in the face of illness, may express **anger** or **frustration**. The caregiver, with patience and understanding, can help channel these emotions by remaining calm and offering explanations or appropriate support, while maintaining an open dialogue.

### Creating a climate of calm

**caregiver** The must also help to create a **climate of calm** within the family, especially when tensions are exacerbated by the patient's critical condition. Through their ability to establish a **calm dialogue**, they can ease family conflicts or misunderstandings that may arise at times of intense stress.

- **Fostering family communication**: The caregiver can facilitate exchanges between family members, creating moments when everyone can express their feelings and participate in decision-making about care. The aim is to strengthen **family unity** at an often fragile time.

## Help with practical aspects of daily life

Caregivers also have a very **practical** role to play in **supporting** families, particularly when it comes to taking care of the patient's daily needs at home, or understanding the gestures to adopt in the course of care.

### Advice on home care

If the patient is cared for at home, families can feel **overwhelmed** by the care required. In such cases, the caregiver is an **invaluable guide**, able to explain the steps to be taken and give practical advice.

- **Settling in** assistance: The caregiver can show families how to help the patient move or reposition to avoid pain or prevent pressure sores. They can teach them the best positions to facilitate breathing or improve the patient's general comfort.

- **Teaching care techniques**: If the family needs to take part in care activities, such as administering medication, using respiratory devices or monitoring vital parameters, the caregiver explains to them **step by step** how to perform these tasks safely and effectively.

**Facilitating organization**

In the context of palliative or long-term care, families often have to juggle medical care, their own professional and personal lives, and sometimes administrative formalities. The caregiver's knowledge of the **care pathway** can guide families towards the resources and **assistance available**.

- **Coordination with the medical team**: The caregiver helps to **coordinate the various parties involved**, so that care runs smoothly and without interruption. They liaise with nurses, doctors and other healthcare professionals to keep the family informed of any changes in the patient's condition or care protocol.

- **Help with managing resources**: They can also inform the family about the help available (financial, social, logistical) and direct them to support services such as **social workers**, **psychologists** or **support groups**.

# Chapter 8

# Emergencies and complications in pneumology

- **Recognizing a respiratory emergency**
  - ○ Acute asthma attack, COPD decompensation, pneumothorax

**Acute asthma attacks, COPD decompensations** and **pneumothorax** are frequent respiratory emergencies requiring rapid, precise management to avoid serious, even life-threatening complications. Although these situations differ in their causes and mechanisms, what they have in common is that they rapidly compromise the patient's **oxygenation** and **ventilation**, leading to acute respiratory distress. Understanding the characteristics of each situation, their warning signs and appropriate treatments is essential for effective intervention.

## Acute asthma attack

**Asthma** is a chronic inflammatory disease of the airways that causes **narrowing of** the bronchial tubes in response to **triggers** such as allergens, respiratory infections, stress or irritants like tobacco smoke. An **acute asthma attack** occurs when the bronchial tubes contract sharply, making breathing difficult and causing intense breathlessness.

### Signs and symptoms

Patients in acute asthma attacks present **characteristic signs** of respiratory distress:

- Severe **dyspnea**, with a sensation of suffocation.
- Audible **sibilance** (wheezing), especially on exhalation.
- Dry **cough**, sometimes accompanied by a feeling of tightness in the chest.
- **Pulling**: using accessory muscles to breathe, resulting in hollowing of the clavicles or abdomen.
- **Cyanosis** (bluish tint of lips and extremities) in severe cases, indicating poor oxygenation.

**Support**

Managing an acute asthma attack requires rapid intervention to prevent the situation from worsening:

1.  **Bronchodilators**: The first line of treatment is bronchodilators, such as inhaled **beta-2 agonists** (salbutamol). These rapidly relax bronchial muscles and reopen the airways.

2.  **Oxygen therapy**: If the patient shows signs of desaturation (SpO2 < 90%), **oxygen** is administered to improve oxygenation. Oxygen saturation monitoring is crucial throughout management.

3.  **Corticosteroids**: If the attack is severe, **corticosteroids** are administered to reduce bronchial inflammation. They are not immediately effective, but help limit the duration and severity of the attack.

4.  **Magnesium sulfate**: In the event of a severe attack that refuses conventional treatment, intravenous administration of **magnesium sulfate** may be considered to promote bronchial relaxation.

5.  **Intubation and ventilation**: In extreme cases, if the seizure does not respond to treatment, intubation and mechanical ventilation may be necessary to avoid respiratory arrest.

# COPD decompensation

**Chronic obstructive pulmonary disease** (COPD) is a progressive disease characterized by inflammation of the bronchial tubes and destruction of the pulmonary alveoli, mainly due to **tobacco smoke**. COPD patients can live with chronic breathlessness, but **decompensation** occurs when a sudden worsening occurs, often in response to infection or exposure to irritants. This leads to a rapid deterioration in respiratory function and requires immediate management.

**Signs and symptoms**

Signs of COPD decompensation include:

- **Increased dyspnea** compared to the patient's basal state. Breathlessness is more intense, even at rest.
- **Sputum**: worsening of cough, with increased quantity and viscosity of secretions. Sputum may be purulent in cases of underlying infection.
- **Wheezing** and **abnormally slow** or **rapid** breathing.
- **Cyanosis** and oxygen **desaturation**, especially in severe cases, where oxygen saturation can fall below 88%.
- **Altered general condition**: intense fatigue, confusion, even drowsiness, due to CO2 retention (hypercapnia).

**Support**

Acute COPD decompensation requires rapid intervention to avoid acute respiratory failure:

1. **Bronchodilators**: As with asthma, bronchodilators are administered to open the airways. **Anticholinergics** )ipratropium bromide) can also be combined with beta-2 agonists to enhance their effect.

2. **Controlled oxygen therapy**: Unlike in asthma, the administration of oxygen in COPD patients must be done with **caution**. Excess oxygen can aggravate hypercapnia in these patients, who depend on hypoxia to stimulate breathing. The aim is to maintain **saturation levels** between 88 and 92%.

3.  **Corticosteroids and antibiotics**: Systemic **corticosteroids** are used to reduce airway inflammation, while **antibiotics** may be prescribed if an infection (pneumonia, infectious bronchitis) is suspected as the cause of decompensation.

4.  **Non-invasive ventilation (NIV)**: In cases of severe hypercapnia, **non-invasive ventilation** (BiPAP) may be required to support ventilation and improve CO2 elimination.

5.  **Intubation**: If decompensation is refractory to treatment, or hypercapnia becomes uncontrollable, intubation with mechanical ventilation may be necessary to stabilize the patient's condition.

## Pneumothorax

**Pneumothorax** occurs when air enters the **pleural cavity**, the space between the lungs and the chest wall, causing partial or total **collapse of** the lung. It can be **spontaneous**, often in young adults with no prior lung pathology, or secondary to underlying lung disease such as COPD or chest trauma. A pneumothorax can rapidly become a life-threatening emergency if it evolves into a **compressive** pneumothorax, a situation where trapped air compresses the lungs and heart, leading to **cardiorespiratory arrest**.

### Signs and symptoms

Signs of pneumothorax include:

-   Sudden, sharp **chest pain**, often on the affected side.
-   **Dyspnea**: sudden shortness of breath, sometimes associated with severe respiratory distress.
-   **Decreased or absent vesicular murmur** (breath sounds) on auscultation on the affected side.

- **Tympany** on percussion of the thorax, due to the presence of air in the pleural cavity.
- In case of compressive pneumothorax: **hypotension, tachycardia**, and **deviation of the trachea** to the opposite side, indicating compression of mediastinal structures.

**Support**

Pneumothorax management depends on the severity and type of pneumothorax.

1. **Oxygen therapy**: In all cases of ,pneumothorax oxygen is administered to improve oxygenation and aid resorption of air in the pleural cavity.

2. **Observation**: If the pneumothorax is small and does not cause severe symptoms, **attentive monitoring** with regular X-rays may be sufficient. Pneumothorax may resolve spontaneously.

3. **Needle exsufflation**: In cases of compressive pneumothorax or severe symptomatic **pneumothorax, emergency exsufflation** with a needle inserted into the second intercostal space enables rapid decompression of the pleural cavity and stabilization of the patient.

4. **Chest drain**: For larger pneumothoraxes or cases requiring prolonged intervention, a **chest drain** is fitted to allow continuous evacuation of air from the pleural cavity. This helps the lung to re-expand.

5. **Surgery**: In recurrent or complicated cases, surgery such as **pleurodesis** (a procedure to glue the two pleural sheets together) may be considered to prevent recurrence.

◦   Warning signs of respiratory distress

The **warning signs of respiratory distress** are essential indicators to recognize early and intervene before the situation worsens. Respiratory distress occurs when the lungs are no longer able to ensure sufficient oxygenation of the blood or adequate removal of carbon dioxide. This can lead to respiratory failure if not treated promptly. Various pathologies can lead to respiratory distress, such as acute asthma, COPD, pneumonia or pneumothorax, and each situation requires an immediate response. Early detection relies on the observation of clinical signs that reflect the body's increased efforts to compensate for the lack of oxygen.

## 1. Dyspnea and changes in breathing

**Dyspnea** (shortness of breath) is often the first sign that a patient is experiencing breathing difficulties. It can occur gradually or suddenly, depending on the underlying pathology.

- **Dyspnea on exertion**: the patient begins to feel disproportionately short of breath for moderate or light exertion. For example, climbing stairs or even walking a few metres may cause abnormal breathlessness.

- **Dyspnea at rest**: As respiratory distress progresses, shortness of breath may occur even at rest. This indicates more advanced **respiratory failure**.

- **Changes in respiratory rate**: **Tachypnea** (rapid breathing) is an early sign. Increased respiratory rate is a response to reduced blood oxygenation. However, in severe cases, **bradypnea** (slowed breathing) may be observed, indicating respiratory decompensation.

- **Shallow breathing**: The patient may breathe more shallowly, with less amplified respiratory movements. This indicates that respiratory effort is becoming ineffective.

199

## 2. Use of accessory muscles

When breathing becomes difficult, the body mobilizes **accessory muscles** to compensate for respiratory insufficiency. These muscles are located in the neck, shoulders and abdomen, and their excessive use is a sign of increased respiratory effort.

- **Intercostal tugging**: The ribs between the intercostal spaces are **hollowed out** during inspiration. This indicates that the respiratory muscles are working hard to inspire.

- **Nostril flapping**: **Nostril** flapping during inspiration is a sign that the body is trying to improve airflow to the lungs.

- **Paradoxical movement of the abdomen**: The diaphragm is the main muscle involved in breathing. In respiratory distress, **paradoxical movements** of the abdomen can be observed, where the abdomen hollows out on inspiration instead of inflating normally.

## 3. Cyanosis

**Cyanosis** is a visual sign that blood oxygenation is insufficient. It manifests as a **bluish discoloration of** the skin, particularly visible around the **lips**, **nail beds** and **earlobes**.

- **Peripheral cyanosis**: first appears in the extremities, such as the fingers and toes. It is an early sign of hypoxia (lack of oxygen in the blood).

- **Central cyanosis**: As hypoxia worsens, cyanosis may also appear on the **upper limbs** and **face**, signaling an even more severe lack of oxygenation.

# 4. Impaired consciousness

**Altered consciousness** is a worrying sign of respiratory distress. Poor oxygenation of the brain rapidly affects cognitive functions.

- **Agitation**: The patient may become agitated or confused, feeling suffocated and instinctively seeking to change position to breathe more easily. This agitation is often linked to the anxiety caused by the sensation of suffocation.

- **Somnolence**: As hypoxia and hypercapnia (excess carbon dioxide in the blood) progress, the patient may become drowsy or display **disturbances of alertness**.

- **Confusion and impaired concentration**: Patients may have difficulty answering questions or following a conversation. **Cognitive impairment** is a sign of advanced cerebral hypoxia.

# 5. Changes in breath sounds

**Breath sounds** can provide valuable clues to respiratory distress. **Auscultatory silence** or abnormal sounds should be regarded as warning signs.

- **Wheezing**: **Wheezing** (often associated with asthma or COPD) indicates airway obstruction. These noises occur mainly during exhalation, when air has difficulty leaving the lungs.

- **Crackling rales**: In cases of pneumonia or pulmonary edema, **crackling** sounds may be heard on inspiration, signaling fluid accumulation in the pulmonary alveoli.

- **Diminished or absent vesicular murmurs**: in cases of pneumothorax or severe bronchial obstruction, **vesicular**

**murmurs** (normal breath sounds) may be diminished or absent on one side of the chest.

# 6. Tachycardia and cardiovascular signs

**Tachycardia** (increased heart rate) is an early response to hypoxia. The body attempts to compensate for reduced oxygenation by increasing blood flow. However, as respiratory distress worsens, more serious cardiovascular signs may appear.

- **Tachycardia**: The heart beats faster in an attempt to deliver more oxygen to the organs. Persistent tachycardia with no improvement in breathing is a sign of worsening.

- **Hypotension**: a drop in blood pressure may occur in severe cases, indicating that the body is in **shock** due to respiratory failure.

# 7. Warning signs in children

Children sometimes present particular signs of respiratory distress that may differ from those observed in adults. It is crucial to pay particular attention to these signs in children.

- **Nostril flapping**: Nostril flapping is very common in children in respiratory distress, and is an early sign of respiratory distress.

- **Breathing moans or grunts**: Infants may make moans or grunts during exhalation, reflecting their efforts to maintain air pressure in the lungs.

- **Subcostal and supraclavicular retractions**: In children, intercostal retractions are often very marked, accompanied by accentuated movements of the abdominal muscles.

- **First aid in pneumology**
  - ○ Setting up emergency oxygen therapy

**Emergency oxygen therapy** is a crucial intervention in cases of **acute respiratory distress**, or when a patient's oxygenation levels drop dangerously low. It immediately improves blood oxygen saturation, stabilizes the patient's condition and prevents serious, even threatening-life complications such as respiratory failure or cardiorespiratory arrest. Emergency oxygen therapy must be implemented rapidly and precisely, taking into account the patient's specific needs and the underlying causes of respiratory distress.

## Indications for emergency oxygen therapy

Emergency oxygen therapy is indicated when the patient shows signs of **hypoxia** (lack of oxygen in the blood) or clinical signs of respiratory distress. These situations include acute illnesses or events such as :

- **Severe asthma attacks**
- **COPD exacerbations**
- **Acute pneumonia**
- **Acute pulmonary edema**
- **Pneumothorax**
- **Thoracic trauma**
- **Cardiorespiratory arrest**

**Signs of hypoxia** requiring immediate oxygen therapy include **oxygen saturation (SpO2) below 90%**, **cyanosis** (bluish discoloration of lips and extremities), **tachycardia**, **altered level of consciousness**, and marked **dyspnea**.

## Initial patient assessment

Before initiating emergency oxygen therapy, a rapid but thorough assessment of the patient's condition is necessary to determine the degree of hypoxia and the amount of oxygen required. The assessment includes:

1.  **Measuring oxygen saturation (SpO2)**: A **pulse oximeter** is used to measure oxygen saturation in the blood. A saturation of less than 90% indicates an immediate need for additional oxygen. In the event of acute respiratory failure, this measurement must be taken continuously to adjust the amount of oxygen administered.

2.  **Respiratory rate**: Patients in respiratory distress often exhibit **tachypnea** (increased respiratory rate), which is a sign of compensation for hypoxia. Worsening tachypnea or slow breathing (bradypnea) is a sign of severity.

3.  **Clinical signs of hypoxia**: **Agitation, confusion, cyanosis, use of accessory muscles** and **tachycardia** or **bradycardia** are major clinical indicators that point to the need for oxygen therapy.

## Choice of oxygenation system

There are several different oxygen delivery devices, each adapted to specific needs in terms of oxygen flow and concentration. The choice of device depends on the severity of respiratory distress and the level of oxygen to be administered.

### 1. Nasal cannula (low-flow oxygen)

**Nasal cannulae** are the simplest and most commonly used device for situations where **moderate oxygen therapy** is required. They deliver oxygen at a flow rate of 1 to 6 liters per minute (L/min), providing an oxygen concentration of 24% to 40%. They are often used in less severe situations, or to maintain adequate oxygen saturation in a stable patient.

- **Indications**: Moderate hypoxemia with saturation between 85% and 92%.
- **Advantages**: Comfortable and easy to tolerate, allowing the patient to speak and eat.

- **Limitations**: Not suitable for patients with severe hypoxemia, as oxygen concentration is relatively low.

## 2. Single oxygen mask

The **simple oxygen mask** is used when nasal cannulae are no longer sufficient to improve oxygenation. It administers oxygen at a flow rate of 5 to 10 L/min, delivering an oxygen concentration of 40 to 60%.

- **Indications**: More severe hypoxemia, when the patient is unable to maintain sufficient saturation with nasal cannula.
- **Benefits**: Delivers a higher level of oxygen than nasal cannula.
- **Limitations**: Less comfortable in the long term, as it covers the nose and mouth.

## 3. High-concentration mask with reservoir (non-rebreathing mask)

The **high-concentration mask with reservoir**, or **non-rebreathing mask**, is used in cases of severe **hypoxia requiring** a high concentration of oxygen. This mask features an oxygen reservoir and a one-way valve that prevents the patient from inhaling exhaled air, thus guaranteeing a **high oxygen concentration**, typically between 60% and 100% at a flow rate of 10 to 15 L/min.

- **Indications**: Severe hypoxemia (SpO2 < 85%), critical situations such as acute pulmonary edema, pneumothorax, or severe COPD decompensation.
- **Benefits**: Provides maximum oxygen concentration, which is crucial in cases of acute respiratory distress.
- **Limitations**: The mask can be uncomfortable to wear for long periods and is not well tolerated by some patients.

### 4. Non-invasive ventilation (NIV)

**Non-invasive ventilation** (NIV) is used for patients suffering from **acute respiratory insufficiency** with hypercapnia (accumulation of CO2), or in cases of cardiac or respiratory insufficiency where simple oxygenation is not sufficient. It delivers oxygen under pressure (by CPAP or BiPAP) to improve respiratory efficiency and reduce respiratory effort.

- **Indications**: COPD decompensation, acute lung edema, acute respiratory distress syndrome (ARDS).
- **Benefits**: Delays or avoids intubation by providing ventilatory support without airway invasion.
- **Limitations**: Requires continuous monitoring, not suitable for unconscious patients or those in respiratory arrest.

### 5. Intubation and mechanical ventilation

In the most severe cases, when non-invasive oxygen therapy is insufficient or the patient can no longer maintain autonomous breathing, **tracheal intubation** and **mechanical ventilation** are necessary.

- **Indications**: Respiratory arrest, shock, coma, or failure of other oxygenation methods.
- **Benefits**: Ensures maximum oxygenation and ventilation, essential in critical situations.
- **Limitations**: Requires specialized skills and intensive management.

## Monitoring during oxygen therapy

Once emergency oxygen therapy has been initiated, **patient monitoring** is crucial to ensure that treatment is effective, and to adjust flow rates if necessary.

1. **Oxygen saturation (SpO2)**: Saturation should be measured continuously to ensure that the patient maintains

an **SpO2 between 92% and 96%** in patients without chronic respiratory failure. In COPD patients, the target saturation is often lower (88-92%) to avoid hypercapnia.

2.  **Respiratory rate and signs of distress**: It is important to continue monitoring **respiratory rate and** clinical signs of distress (cyanosis, draught, use of accessory muscles) to assess the effectiveness of oxygenation.

3.  **Blood gases**: In cases of severe hypoxia or suspected hypercapnia, arterial **blood gas analysis** is often necessary to assess the patient's oxygenation (PaO2) and ventilation (PaCO2), and to adjust the management strategy.

4.  **Side effects of oxygen therapy**: Although oxygen is vital, excess oxygen can lead to undesirable effects, such as hypercapnia in **COPD** patients, or **oxygen toxicity** in the event of prolonged exposure to high concentrations. Particular vigilance is therefore required to avoid over-oxygenating patients.

      ◦    Positioning the patient in distress

**Positioning the patient** in a situation of **respiratory distress** is a key element in managing such an emergency. Adopting the right posture can relieve breathlessness, facilitate breathing and improve oxygenation. It's a non-invasive but often highly effective intervention to help the patient return to more comfortable breathing before or in addition to other medical measures, such as oxygen administration. The optimum position depends on the severity of the respiratory distress, the underlying cause and the patient's comfort.

# Objectives of positioning in respiratory distress

The aim of positioning is to :

- **Improve lung expansion** by facilitating movement of the ribcage and diaphragm.
- **Reduce respiratory effort** by using accessory muscles more efficiently.
- **Improve oxygenation** by reducing lung compression and facilitating gas exchange.
- **Relieve anxiety** by adopting a position that reduces the sensation of suffocation.

# Recommended positions in case of respiratory distress

### 1. Sitting or semi-seated position (Fowler position)

The **semi-seated** position (or **Fowler position**) is one of the most widely used to relieve breathlessness in respiratory distress. The patient is placed in a reclined position, at an angle of 30 to 45 degrees, or more if necessary.

- **Advantages**: In the semi-seated position, the **diaphragm** descends better during inspiration, allowing **the lungs to expand** more fully. This posture also reduces compression of the lungs by the abdominal organs. It also facilitates the use of **accessory muscles** for breathing, which can reduce respiratory effort.

- **Indications**: This **position** is indicated for patients with chronic respiratory diseases such as **COPD, pneumonia**, or **acute asthma attacks**. It is also beneficial for patients with **pulmonary edema** or **heart failure**.

- **Precautions**: To avoid pressure sores in bedridden patients, it's essential to adjust their position regularly. A support under the knees can also be used to limit the risk of slipping in bed, which could cause discomfort.

## 2. Seated position with support (tripod position)

The **tripod position** is often instinctively adopted by patients in **severe respiratory distress**, as it effectively relieves breathlessness. In this position, the patient is seated, leaning forward, with **forearms resting on** a table, bed or lap.

- **Benefits**: This posture **mobilizes the accessory muscles** (neck, shoulder and chest muscles) and promotes thoracic expansion. It also reduces pressure on the **diaphragm**, making breathing easier. Leaning forward reduces the sensation of suffocation and helps calm anxiety linked to respiratory distress.

- **Indications**: This **position** is particularly effective for patients suffering from **decompensating COPD, asthma attacks** or other conditions where thoracic expansion is limited. It is also often used instinctively by patients suffering from **pneumothorax**, as it reduces chest pain by decreasing pressure on the chest.

- **Precautions**: The caregiver must ensure that the patient is properly supported to avoid excessive fatigue, as remaining in this position for too long can become uncomfortable. Cushions or a stable surface can be used to support the arms.

## 3. Lying on your side (lateral decubitus)

The **lateral position** (or **lateral decubitus**) can be beneficial for patients who cannot tolerate the sitting position, or who present with unilateral pathology, such as **pneumonia** or **pneumothorax**.

- **Advantages**: Placing the patient on the **unaffected side** allows the healthy lung to ventilate better, promoting optimal gas exchange. It also reduces pressure on the diseased lung. This position is more comfortable for some patients with chest or abdominal pain.

- **Indications**: This posture is particularly indicated for patients with **pneumothorax** or **unilateral lobar pneumonia**, as it helps optimize ventilation of the functional lung.

- **Precautions**: It is essential to support the patient correctly with cushions to avoid prolonged pressure on the support points, which could lead to pressure sores.

## 4. Prone position

The **prone position**, or **proning**, involves placing the patient on his or her stomach. This position is mainly used in patients with severe respiratory distress, particularly in the context of **acute respiratory distress syndrome (ARDS)**.

- **Advantages**: This position promotes **better perfusion of the posterior parts of the lungs,** which are often better ventilated due to gravity. This improves the patient's overall oxygenation, as the areas dependent on the lungs are less compressed by the abdominal organs and rib cage.

- **Indications**: **Prone positioning** is mainly used in the hospital setting for **mechanically ventilated** patients, but can also be used as a preventive measure for certain ARDS patients in intensive care. It has become particularly important in the management of **acute respiratory failure** in cases such as COVID-19.

- **Precautions**: This position can be uncomfortable and requires careful monitoring to prevent complications, such as skin lesions, nerve compressions or difficulties in maintaining an unobstructed airway. It is generally used in rotation with other positions.

# Other important considerations

## 1. Monitor anxiety

Patients in respiratory distress are often highly **anxious**, and this anxiety can exacerbate their difficulty in breathing. Adopting a position that **reassures** them and reduces the sensation of suffocation is crucial to calming their agitation. The caregiver should encourage adapted **breathing techniques**, such as pursed-lip breathing, to help control panic.

## 2. Maintain a calm environment

A calm, soothing environment also helps to relieve anxiety and improve tolerance to comfort positions. Limiting **stressful stimuli** such as excessive noise and offering psychological support can help improve the effectiveness of positional treatment.

## 3. Adapting positions to treatments

When respiratory assistance devices are used (oxygen spectacles, oxygen masks or non-invasive ventilation), the patient's position must **facilitate their use** without interfering with care. For example, when seated or in a tripod position, it is essential that the oxygen therapy device remains snug and comfortable to ensure optimal oxygenation.

- **Collaborate with the team in emergency situations**
  - Everyone's role in respiratory resuscitation

**Respiratory resuscitation** is a critical intervention in the event of cardiopulmonary arrest or severe respiratory failure. Each member of the healthcare team has a clearly defined role to play in ensuring rapid, effective care. Optimum coordination between the various players is crucial to maximize the patient's chances of survival. Here are the **main roles** of each player in respiratory resuscitation, generally based on protocols such as **Advanced Cardiovascular Life Support** (ACLS) and international resuscitation guidelines.

# 1. The team leader (doctor or senior nurse)

The **team leader** coordinates the entire resuscitation team. He or she is often an **emergency physician**, an **anesthesiologist** or a **senior nurse** qualified in advanced resuscitation techniques.

**Main roles :**

- **Decision-making**: Directs the entire resuscitation, making critical decisions on actions to be taken, such as when to administer drugs, intubate the patient or change ventilation methods.
- **Team supervision**: Ensures proper coordination of each team member, distributes roles if this has not yet been done, and ensures that each task is carried out correctly.
- **Communication**: Keeps an overview of the situation, communicates clearly and ensures that other team members understand instructions. He may also relay information to other medical teams or to the patient's relatives after resuscitation.
- **Patient assessment**: Continuously assesses the patient's condition, based on vital parameters, responses to interventions and test results (electrocardiogram, saturation, etc.).

## 2. The cardiac massager

The **cardiac masseur** is often a caregiver, nurse or member trained in basic resuscitation techniques. They play a vital role in maintaining blood flow to vital organs until breathing and heart rhythm are restored.

**Main roles :**

- **Performing chest compressions**: He performs high-quality **chest compressions** as recommended: a depth of 5 to 6 cm in adults, at a frequency of 100 to 120 compressions per minute, while allowing complete re-expansion of the chest between each compression.
- **Rotating with another caregiver**: Chest compressions are exhausting, and the cardiac masseur must rotate with another team member every two minutes to maintain the effectiveness of the compressions.
- **Coordination with ventilation**: He must ensure that compressions are synchronized with ventilation if the latter is in progress. If the patient is intubated, compressions and ventilation can be performed independently of each other.

## 3. The fan or ventilation manager

The **ventilator**, often a **nurse anesthetist** or **nurse trained in** resuscitation, manages the patient's airway and ventilation.

**Main roles :**

- **Ensuring ventilation**: He ensures ventilation by means of a **self-filling bag** (AMBU) connected to a source of oxygen, or by using a mechanical ventilator if the patient is intubated.

- **Airway management**: He may use an **oropharyngeal cannula** to keep the airway clear, or be responsible for **tracheal intubation** in cases of prolonged respiratory failure, or if intubation is decided by the team leader.
- **Checking ventilation efficiency**: monitors the patient's chest expansion to ensure that ventilation is efficient and that there are no airway leaks or obstructions.
- **Coordination with the cardiac masseur**: He must coordinate ventilation with chest compressions when there is no intubation, administering two insufflations for every 30 compressions as part of **Basic Life Support** (BLS).

## 4. The nurse in charge of medication

A **nurse** trained in emergency care prepares and administers the drugs needed for resuscitation.

**Main roles :**

- **Medication preparation**: He prepares the drugs used during resuscitation (such as **adrenaline**, **amiodarone**, or other agents depending on the clinical situation and current protocols).
- **Medication administration**: Administers medications under the supervision of the team leader, often by intravenous (IV) or intraosseous (IO) route if IV access is not possible.
- **Medication response monitoring**: Monitors the effects of medication on the patient's vital signs (heart rate, oxygen saturation, blood pressure) and informs the team leader of any response or lack of response.

# 5. The person in charge of monitoring and defibrillation

Another caregiver, usually a **nurse, technician** or **doctor**, is responsible for monitoring vital parameters and managing **defibrillation** if necessary.

**Main roles :**

- **Electrocardiogram (ECG)**: Places and monitors ECG electrodes to check the patient's heart rhythm and identify arrhythmias or cardiac arrest requiring an electric shock.
- **Defibrillation**: If the patient presents with an arrhythmia treatable by **electric shock** (such as **ventricular fibrillation** or **pulseless ventricular tachycardia**), the defibrillation manager prepares the defibrillator and administers the shock in synchronization with other team members.
- **Data analysis**: Between each resuscitation cycle, he analyzes the monitoring and defibrillator data, and reports to the team leader on the evolution of the cardiac rhythm and the effectiveness of the interventions.

# 6. The pathways manager (nurse or doctor)

The **access manager** is responsible for obtaining venous or intraosseous access for medication and fluid administration.

**Main roles :**

- **Placing venous lines**: He places a **peripheral venous line** to administer emergency medication. If this proves difficult, he may consider **intraosseous access** to ensure rapid drug administration.
- **Fluid administration**: If necessary, he prepares and administers **filling solutions** (such as saline or Ringer's lactate) in the event of shock or severe dehydration.

215

## 7. Relay with family and friends (senior team member)

A **doctor** or a senior member of the nursing team is usually responsible for **relaying information to family and friends**. Their role is to inform relatives of the situation and answer any questions they may have.

**Main roles :**

- **Informing loved ones**: Communicates with the patient's loved ones, informing them of the patient's condition and ongoing interventions, while offering emotional support.
- **Managing expectations**: Clearly and empathetically explains the issues involved in resuscitation and, where appropriate, the chances of success or failure, depending on the progress of resuscitation.
- **Accompaniment**: If resuscitation is unsuccessful, he accompanies relatives through this difficult time, explaining the situation and providing psychological support.

　　　　　○　　Feedback and learning after an emergency

**Feedback and learning after an emergency** are essential steps in improving the quality of care and enhancing the competence of medical teams. After an emergency intervention, whether cardiopulmonary resuscitation, anaphylactic shock or acute respiratory distress, it is crucial to take time to analyze the actions taken, assess their effectiveness and identify areas for improvement. This phase of collective reflection, often referred to as **debriefing**, not only enables lessons to be learned from the experience, but also strengthens team cohesion and improves practices for future situations.

# The importance of feedback after an emergency

Feedback, when well conducted, plays a crucial role in the progression of professional skills, particularly in environments where emergency situations are frequent and unpredictable. This process enables :

- **Analyze individual and collective performance**: Debriefing enables us to assess individual performance, as well as team dynamics. Understanding how roles were distributed, how communication was managed, and whether protocols were respected, provides valuable lessons for improving future interventions.

- **Identify areas for improvement**: During an emergency, certain interventions can be carried out under pressure, sometimes with errors or inaccuracies. Feedback helps to **highlight errors** or moments of doubt, so that we can understand their cause and avoid their recurrence.

- **Reinforce technical and non-technical skills**: In addition to assessing technical skills (such as airway management or chest compressions), feedback can be used to work on **non-technical skills**, such as **communication**, **leadership**, **decision-making under pressure**, and **stress management**.

- **Preserving team cohesion**: debriefing also provides a space for expressing **emotions** and **feelings** after sometimes trying situations, especially when they are marked by a fatal outcome. This strengthens **solidarity** between team members and eases any tensions.

## The debriefing process: a key learning tool

**Debriefing** is the most structured form of feedback after an emergency. It generally takes place in the minutes or hours following the event, and involves all team members who took part

217

in the response. To be effective, it must respect several fundamental principles:

## 1. Creating an environment of trust

For debriefing to be constructive, it's essential to create an **environment** of **trust**, where everyone feels free to express their ideas, successes and mistakes, without fear of judgment. The aim is not to point fingers, but to learn together.

- **Encourage participation**: All team members, from senior doctors to caregivers, should be encouraged to share their impressions. A diversity of viewpoints is invaluable for gaining an overall vision of the intervention.

- **Avoid judgment**: Comments should be **constructive** and aimed at improvement, avoiding any accusatory tone. The team leader or debriefing facilitator must take care to maintain a benevolent and respectful discussion.

## 2. Analysis of key actions

Once a climate of trust has been established, the debriefing focuses on a **detailed analysis of** the **actions** taken during the emergency. This phase identifies what worked well and what could have been improved.

- **Examination of procedures**: Compliance with protocols is a central element. We analyze whether emergency care procedures have been correctly followed, whether medications have been administered in a timely manner, and whether technical gestures (chest compressions, intubation, defibrillation) have been performed effectively and in a timely manner.

- **Evaluation of roles and communication**: Particular attention is paid to the **distribution of roles and** the quality of **communication** during the intervention. Poor task allocation or misunderstood instructions can lead to delays or errors. Identifying these problems helps us to improve for future interventions.

### 3. Discussion of difficulties encountered

During an emergency, **unexpected difficulties** can arise, whether technical, human or organizational. Feedback enables these to be examined in detail.

- **Technical problems**: Some equipment may not function as expected, or malfunctions may occur. For example, a problem with an oxygen mask or difficulty in obtaining a venous access line. These difficulties need to be discussed with a view to finding corrective solutions (maintenance, additional training).

- **Stress management**: The **emotional impact of** emergency situations can affect caregivers' performance. Recognizing these stressful moments and discussing them openly helps to identify **stress management strategies**, such as breathing training or mutual support during the intervention.

### 4. Identify areas for improvement

The debriefing should conclude by highlighting **areas for improvement** for future interventions. This includes implementing **concrete strategies** to avoid mistakes, strengthen weak points and capitalize on successes.

- **Skills enhancement**: If technical shortcomings are identified, it may be advisable to organize **additional training** or **simulation exercises** to reinforce skills. For example, a team with recurring intubation difficulties could plan specific training sessions.

- **Strengthen coordination**: If communication problems have been identified, it may be beneficial to review communication protocols in emergency situations, or to organize practical exercises to improve the fluidity of exchanges within the team.

## Continuous learning and feedback

Beyond immediate debriefing, the experience of an emergency must be part of a **continuous learning** process. Each situation is an opportunity to enrich collective know-how and improve the quality of care.

### 1. Integrate lessons into daily practice

The lessons learned from a debriefing must be integrated into daily practice. This may involve **revising protocols**, improving care procedures, or disseminating **best practices** within the team.

- **Updating protocols**: If an intervention has revealed a flaw or ambiguity in existing procedures, it is essential to update protocols to ensure that future interventions are smoother and better organized.

- **Sharing experience**: Learning after an emergency should not be restricted to the participants. Feedback can be shared with the whole medical or paramedical team to spread the lessons learned and prevent other teams from encountering the same difficulties.

## 2. Organize regular training sessions

Learning doesn't just happen in real-life emergencies. It's important to maintain **regular** team **training** through emergency **simulations**, practical workshops and ongoing training.

- **Emergency simulations**: Organizing **simulation scenarios** enables the team to prepare for different critical situations. These simulations reproduce real emergency conditions, using mannequins or high-tech devices, and are followed by structured debriefings.

- **Feedback**: Real-life emergency situations can be used as a basis for training. Recreating scenarios based on past events helps to reinforce skills in specific problem cases.

## 3. Ensuring the mental health of caregivers

It's essential not to overlook the **emotional impact of** emergency care on caregivers. Some situations can be particularly difficult, especially if they result in patient failure or loss.

- **Psychological support**: Providing caregivers with **psychological support** helps them deal with the stress and emotions associated with emergency care. Providing a space to talk about feelings experienced during a difficult resuscitation or stressful situation helps prevent burn-out.

- **Encouraging mutual support**: The post-emergency period is also an opportunity to strengthen **mutual support** within the team. Supporting colleagues, expressing gratitude for a job well done, and sharing successes and failures all help to build solidarity and team spirit.

# Chapter 9

# Respiratory and geriatric care

- **Management of elderly patients with respiratory diseases**
  - Fragility of the elderly in the face of pulmonary infections

The **fragility of the elderly in the face of pulmonary infections** is a major public health issue, particularly as the population ages. With age, the body undergoes numerous physiological changes that weaken the immune system, lung capacity and response to infection. These changes make the elderly more vulnerable to **lung infections**, such as **pneumonia**, **bronchitis** and **exacerbations of COPD** (chronic obstructive pulmonary disease). These infections, often commonplace in young adults, can lead to serious or even fatal complications in the elderly. Understanding this fragility will enable us to better prevent, diagnose and treat lung infections in this at-risk population.

# 1. Ageing and reduced immune defences

One of the main factors making the elderly vulnerable to lung infections is the **aging of the immune system**, a phenomenon known as **immunosenescence**. With age, the immune system's ability to identify and combat pathogens such as viruses and bacteria diminishes.

**Impaired innate and adaptive immunity**

- **Innate immunity**: The body's first line of defense, which includes physical barriers such as **mucous membranes** and immune cells like **macrophages**, becomes less effective. In the elderly, the production of protective mucus in the respiratory tract may diminish, making it easier for pathogens to invade.

- **Adaptive immunity**: with age, the number and function of **T** and **B lymphocytes** are altered. These cells play an essential role in the specific recognition of infections and the production of antibodies. As a result, the immune response is slower and less effective in the elderly, increasing the risk of contracting lung infections and developing severe forms.

**Lower vaccine response**

**Vaccine response** is also less effective in the elderly. For example, although the **influenza** and **pneumococcal** vaccines are recommended for this population, the protection they offer is often reduced compared to younger adults. This phenomenon of low vaccine response is compounded by the natural vulnerability of the elderly to respiratory infections.

# 2. Age-related changes in lung function

As we age, **lung function** undergoes anatomical and physiological changes that make the lungs less able to defend themselves against infection. Reduced lung elasticity and weakened respiratory muscles exacerbate this situation.

**Decreased lung capacity**

**Aging lungs** gradually lose their ability to expand and contract efficiently. **Alveoli lose** elasticity, limiting gas exchange. This reduction in lung capacity affects ventilation and the ability to effectively expel inhaled pathogens or bronchial secretions, favoring their accumulation and the onset of infections.

**Weakness of respiratory muscles**

**Respiratory muscles**, such as the diaphragm, weaken with age. This reduces the effectiveness of **coughing**, a natural defense mechanism for expelling secretions or foreign particles from the lungs. In an elderly person, an ineffective cough promotes mucus retention in the bronchi, creating a breeding ground for bacterial proliferation and infection.

# 3. Frequent co-morbidities

The elderly often suffer from **chronic co-morbidities**, which increase their vulnerability to pulmonary infections. These conditions, whether respiratory or not, impair their general condition and diminish their ability to cope with a new infection.

### COPD and heart failure

**Chronic respiratory diseases**, such as **COPD** (chronic obstructive pulmonary disease), are common among the elderly. The lungs, already weakened by this disease, are more likely to develop **exacerbations** during lung infections, making recovery longer and more difficult.

In addition, diseases such as **heart failure** affect blood circulation and oxygen supply to tissues, compounding the impact of a pulmonary infection. The interaction between these different pathologies further weakens the body, increasing the risk of **complications** such as acute respiratory failure or septic shock.

### Diabetes and immune deficiency

**Diabetes**, also common in the elderly, reduces the body's ability to fight infections, including lung infections. Diabetes weakens the immune system and impairs the functions of macrophages and neutrophils, cells essential for destroying pathogens. In addition, diabetic patients are more likely to develop more serious infections and complications, such as pulmonary abscesses or purulent pleurisy.

# 4. Nutritional fragility and sarcopenia

**Malnutrition** and **sarcopenia** (loss of muscle mass) are common in the elderly, and play an aggravating role in their susceptibility to pulmonary infections.

### Impact of malnutrition on immunity

Malnutrition, particularly in **proteins** and **vitamins** (such as vitamin D and vitamin C), further weakens the immune system. Inadequate nutritional status reduces antibody production and the body's ability to repair lung tissue damaged by infection. This increases the **morbidity** and **mortality** of lung infections in the elderly.

### Sarcopenia and respiratory weakness

**Sarcopenia** leads to a general loss of muscular strength, including in the **respiratory muscles**. This weakness reduces the ability of the elderly to expel pulmonary secretions by coughing, leading to **stagnation of secretions** and the onset of superinfections. Physical deconditioning, often observed in the frail elderly, exacerbates this situation.

## 5. Increased risk of complications

In the elderly, lung infections, whether viral or bacterial in origin, often lead to **serious complications**. These complications can manifest themselves in the lungs, but also have systemic repercussions on the whole body.

### Respiratory complications

Respiratory complications are common in the elderly. Bacterial **pneumonia** can lead to **pulmonary edema** or **acute respiratory failure**, requiring hospitalization or even intubation and mechanical ventilation. Pulmonary infections can also cause severe **exacerbations** in COPD patients, leading to prolonged hospitalization and an increased risk of mortality.

### Systemic complications

Pulmonary infections can also cause **systemic complications** in the elderly. For example, severe pulmonary infection can progress to **sepsis** (generalized inflammatory reaction) or **septic shock**, potentially fatal conditions requiring intensive care. The interaction between infection and chronic co-morbidities (heart failure, diabetes) exacerbates these complications.

## 6. The importance of prevention

Given the increased vulnerability of the elderly to lung infections, **prevention** plays a vital role in reducing the risk and severity of infections. Prevention is based on a number of factors:

### Vaccination

**Vaccination** against influenza and **pneumococcus** is essential to reduce the incidence and severity of respiratory infections in the elderly. Although vaccine efficacy is reduced in this population due to immunosenescence, vaccination remains a key means of preventing serious complications.

### Hygiene and environment

Elderly people living in institutions, such as nursing homes, are exposed to an increased risk of transmitting infections. **Rigorous** hand **hygiene**, surface disinfection and reduced contact with sick people are important measures for limiting the transmission of respiratory infections.

### Maintaining nutrition and physical activity

Maintaining good nutritional status in the elderly, with an adequate intake of **proteins**, **vitamins** and **trace elements**, is essential to support the immune system and prevent infections. In addition, encouraging **regular physical activity** helps preserve muscle strength, including that of the respiratory muscles, which helps maintain good lung capacity.

○ Adapting care to senility and dependence

**Adapting care to senility and dependency** represents a major challenge in the care of the elderly. As they age, many people develop cognitive and physical disorders that impair their autonomy, their ability to understand and follow instructions, and their ability to express their needs. **Senility**, a term often used to describe advanced forms of **dementia** or cognitive decline, further complicates care management. As for **dependency**, whether partial or total, it requires assistance with the acts of daily living and increased support from caregivers. Adapting care to these situations ensures maximum **well-being** and **quality of life** for patients, while respecting their dignity.

## 1. Understanding senility and its implications

**Senility**, often linked to diseases such as **Alzheimer's** or other forms of **dementia**, affects the patient's **memory**, **reasoning** and **cognitive abilities**. This leads to difficulties in understanding medical instructions, cooperating in care or expressing pain and discomfort. Patients may also display **behavioral disorders**, such as agitation, aggression or apathy, further complicating management.

### Communication and compliance difficulties

One of the main challenges facing caregivers in the face of senility is **communication**. Patients may have difficulty understanding simple instructions, remembering what they are told or expressing their needs clearly.

- **Adapting communication**: It's essential to use **simple**, clear **language**, avoiding medical jargon. Gently repeating instructions and making sure the patient has understood is a necessary approach. For example, when administering a treatment, it can be helpful to give one instruction at a time, explaining each step calmly. In addition, the use of **gestures** or **visual cues** can reinforce understanding.

- **Pay close attention to non-verbal cues**: Senile patients may not be able to communicate their pain or discomfort verbally. Caregivers need to pay particular attention to **non-verbal signs**, such as facial expressions, mood changes, or changes in behavior (agitation, refusal to eat), which may indicate a need for medical intervention.

### Taking behavioral problems into account

Senility is often accompanied by **behavioral disorders** such as anxiety, aggression or confusion, which can make caregiving difficult. These disorders are often exacerbated by a lack of understanding of the care provided, or by the medical environment, which is perceived as threatening.

- **Creating a soothing environment**: To minimize anxiety and agitation, it's essential to create a **calm, familiar environment**. This includes **visual cues** (photos, personal objects) that help the patient feel secure and reduce confusion. **Soft lighting** and the absence of sudden noises can also soothe the patient.

- **Adopt an empathetic, patient approach**: Caregivers need to show **patience** and **empathy**, understanding that aggressive or withdrawn reactions are often manifestations of fear or frustration linked to a lack of understanding of the situation. Taking the time to reassure patients, even if this means repeating the same explanations several times, is crucial to gaining their cooperation.

## 2. Adapting care to physical dependence

**Physical dependence** is common among the elderly, due to progressive loss of **mobility** and **muscle strength**, or the onset of chronic illnesses such as osteoarthritis, stroke or COPD. This loss of autonomy requires care adaptations to help the patient carry out the acts of daily life, while maintaining dignity and a sense of autonomy.

**Assistance with everyday tasks**

Dependent patients often need help with **hygiene, meals** and **mobility**. This assistance must be adapted to their physical condition, while encouraging them to participate actively, even partially, in order to maintain a minimum of autonomy.

- **Toileting and personal hygiene**: When patients are no longer able to wash themselves, caregivers must intervene **in** a delicate and respectful manner, taking care to **preserve privacy**. It's a good idea to involve the patient as much as possible in the gestures he or she can still perform, for example by giving him or her a glove so that he or she can wash the accessible parts himself or herself. This maintains his residual autonomy and sense of control.

- **Meals and nutrition**: Dependent people may need help with eating, especially if they have muscle weakness or tremors. The caregiver must offer an **adapted diet**, often broken down into small portions and easy to chew. It is important to encourage patients to feed themselves if they are able to do so, even using **adapted utensils** (light, non-slip) that make taking food easier. The presence of swallowing disorders in dependent patients must also be monitored to prevent false routes.

**Mobilization and prevention of complications related to immobility**

In dependent patients, the **risk of complications** linked to immobility, such as **bedsores, muscular contractures** and **urinary tract infections**, is high. Adapting care therefore means ensuring **regular mobilization** and preventing these complications.

- **Change position regularly**: To prevent pressure sores, it's crucial to regularly change the patient's position, using **special cushions** or **mattresses** to relieve pressure points. This can include gentle limb movements to prevent contractures and maintain muscle flexibility.

- **Encouraging mobility**: Even very dependent people need to be encouraged to move, even minimally. Passive or active exercises, accompanied by a caregiver or physiotherapist, can help prevent total loss of mobility and stimulate blood circulation.

- **Monitoring physiological needs**: Immobility also increases the risk of **urinary retention** and **urinary tract infections**. It is therefore important to monitor urination and encourage the patient to use the toilet regularly, or to mobilize the bowels if bedridden. The use of specific treatments (such as catheters or absorbent devices) must be carried out with care and respect for the patient's dignity.

# 3. Maintain quality of life and psychological well-being

**Dependency** and **senility** can lead to a **sense of loss of** control, **low** self-esteem and **social isolation**, seriously affecting patients' quality of life. Care must therefore also aim to maintain **psychological well-being** and **self-esteem** by reinforcing social ties and offering moments of interaction and cognitive stimulation.

### Encourage participation in social and recreational activities

Dependent or senile patients can tend to withdraw into themselves, especially when they have difficulty communicating or getting around. It's important to **stimulate their interest in** activities that give them pleasure and well-being.

- **Adapted activities**: Activities must be adapted to the patient's cognitive and physical level. For example, simple memory games, reading or music sessions can be beneficial for senile patients. **Manual activities**, such as drawing or gardening, can also improve morale while preserving certain motor functions.

- **Maintaining social relationships**: It's important to foster **communication with loved ones** and maintain regular **social interactions**, whether with nursing staff or other residents in care facilities. These interactions help combat isolation, a source of **depression** and **anxiety** in dependent elderly people.

**Taking individuality and preferences into account**

Personalized care is essential to respect patients' **dignity** and **choice**. This means taking into account their **lifestyle**, **preferences** and **values**.

- **Respect patient preferences**: When a patient expresses preferences for certain aspects of his or her care, such as eating habits, choice of clothing, or grooming routines, it's important to respect them as much as possible. This helps preserve the patient's **identity** and psychological **autonomy**.

- **Involving patients in decisions**: Even in cases of advanced senility or dependency, patients should be **involved in decisions** concerning their own care, wherever possible. This strengthens their sense of control over their lives and enhances their **well-being**.

- **Particularities of respiratory pathologies in the geriatric patient**
  - COPD, respiratory failure and pneumonia in the elderly

**COPD** (chronic obstructive pulmonary disease), **respiratory failure** and **pneumonia** are three serious respiratory conditions that frequently affect the elderly. These pathologies, although different in origin and mechanism, are often interconnected in the elderly due to aging lungs, diminished immune defenses and the presence of co-morbidities. The combination of these conditions can rapidly lead to a deterioration in general health, making their management more complex and increasing the risk of severe complications.

# COPD in the elderly

**COPD** is a chronic respiratory disease characterized by progressive and irreversible obstruction of the airways. It is mainly caused by prolonged exposure to irritants such as **tobacco smoke**, but can also be linked to exposure to environmental or occupational pollutants. In the elderly, COPD is often associated with a long smoking history, and may be diagnosed late, as its symptoms are sometimes confused with the normal signs of aging.

### Mechanisms of COPD

COPD results from two main pathological processes: **chronic bronchitis** and **emphysema**. Chronic bronchitis leads to inflammation and thickening of the bronchial walls, with excessive mucus production obstructing the airways. Emphysema, on the other hand, causes destruction of the pulmonary alveoli, reducing the surface area available for gas exchange.

In the elderly, the natural loss of lung elasticity due to aging exacerbates these processes, further reducing lung capacity and increasing **dyspnoea** (shortness of breath). What's more, COPD is often accompanied by **chronic hypoxia** (low oxygen levels in the blood), which affects quality of life and exercise tolerance.

**Symptoms and complications of COPD**

COPD symptoms are often more pronounced in the elderly and include:

- **Dyspnea** on exertion, then at rest as the disease progresses.
- **Chronic** productive **cough**, often more frequent in the morning.
- Frequent **expectoration**, with excess mucus in the respiratory tract.
- **Wheezing** and tightness in the chest.

Complications of COPD in the elderly include acute **exacerbations**, often triggered by respiratory infections such as pneumonia. These exacerbations manifest as a sudden worsening of symptoms, increased difficulty in breathing and a rapid fall in oxygen saturation. These episodes may require emergency hospitalization and, in severe cases, lead to acute **respiratory failure**.

# Respiratory failure in the elderly

**Respiratory failure** occurs when the lungs are no longer able to ensure adequate gas exchange, resulting in hypoxia (lack of oxygen) and sometimes hypercapnia (excess carbon dioxide). In the elderly, this failure can be caused by **COPD**, but also by other respiratory pathologies, such as pneumonia, emphysema, or the after-effects of vascular accidents.

235

**Types of respiratory failure**

There are two main types of respiratory failure:

1.  **Acute respiratory failure**: This occurs suddenly, often during an acute exacerbation of COPD, lung infection or other respiratory condition. It is characterized by a rapid fall in oxygen saturation and an inability to maintain adequate oxygenation without urgent medical intervention.

2.  **Chronic respiratory insufficiency**: This type of insufficiency sets in gradually, particularly in COPD sufferers. Breathing becomes increasingly difficult over time, and chronic hypoxia leads to complications such as fatigue, pulmonary hypertension and right heart failure (cor pulmonale).

In the elderly, respiratory failure may also be precipitated by increased fragility of the respiratory muscles, making spontaneous ventilation less efficient. This weakness, combined with an age-related reduction in lung capacity, increases the risk of decompensation.

**Management of respiratory failure**

Managing respiratory failure in the elderly requires a tailored, often multidisciplinary, approach to stabilize the situation and avoid complications.

*   **Oxygen therapy**: used to correct hypoxia and improve oxygenation of vital organs. In cases of chronic respiratory insufficiency linked to COPD, **long-term oxygen therapy** may be necessary.

- **Non-invasive ventilation**: For patients suffering from acute or chronic hypercapnic respiratory failure, **non-invasive ventilation** (such as CPAP or BiPAP) is often used to reduce respiratory effort and improve gas exchange.

- **Pharmacological treatments**: **Bronchodilators, corticosteroids** and **mucolytic drugs** are frequently prescribed to reduce airway obstruction and relieve symptoms.

## Pneumonia in the elderly

**Pneumonia** is an infection of the lungs caused by bacteria, viruses or fungi. It is particularly common and dangerous in the elderly, due to their weakened immune systems and co-morbidities. **Community-acquired** and **nosocomial** (hospital-acquired) **pneumonia** are major causes of morbidity and mortality in the elderly.

### Risk factors for pneumonia in the elderly

The elderly are more vulnerable to pneumonia for several reasons:

- **Weakening of the immune system**: With age, the immune response becomes less effective, making respiratory infections more frequent and more serious.
- **Presence of co-morbidities**: Chronic conditions such as diabetes, heart failure, COPD or kidney disease further weaken the ability to fight lung infections.
- **Impaired respiratory function**: Decreased respiratory muscle strength and loss of lung elasticity limit the ability to efficiently evacuate secretions, thus promoting infection.
- **Immobility and prolonged bed rest**: Elderly people who are immobilized, especially in hospitals or nursing homes,

are more likely to develop pneumonia due to the accumulation of secretions in the lungs.

## Symptoms and complications of pneumonia

In the elderly, symptoms of pneumonia may be atypical and less obvious than in young adults. Classic signs such as cough, fever and chest pain may be absent or less pronounced. Instead, we may observe:

- **Mental confusion** or **disorientation**, which may be the first signs of pulmonary infection in the elderly.
- **Extreme fatigue** and **general weakness**, often exacerbated by loss of appetite and dehydration.
- **Dyspnea** or shortness of breath, even at rest.
- **Worsening of co-morbidities**, such as COPD exacerbation or heart failure.

Complications of pneumonia in the elderly can be serious, not least because of their reduced ability to fight infection. They include:

- **Acute respiratory failure**, often requiring hospitalization.
- **Sepsis**, a systemic inflammatory response to infection that can lead to septic shock.
- **Pleuresis**, an accumulation of fluid around the lungs that makes breathing more difficult.

## Treatment of pneumonia in the elderly

The treatment of pneumonia in the elderly relies on rapid management tailored to the patient's general condition.

- **Antibiotics**: In cases of bacterial pneumonia, **antibiotics** are essential and must be administered promptly. In the elderly, it is crucial to monitor responses to treatment, as pharmacokinetics can be altered by age and comorbidities.

- **Oxygen therapy**: As with respiratory failure, oxygen therapy is often used to improve oxygenation in patients with severe pneumonia.

- **Hydration and nutritional support**: The general condition of the elderly can rapidly deteriorate in the event of pneumonia. It is therefore essential to ensure that patients are well **hydrated** and receive adequate nutritional support.

- **Respiratory rehabilitation**: After the acute phase of pneumonia, respiratory **rehabilitation** exercises **may** be recommended to improve lung function and prevent recurrence of infection.

         ○    Mobility problems and impact on breathing

**Mobility problems** and their repercussions on **breathing** are a major issue, particularly for the elderly or those suffering from chronic pathologies. Reduced mobility, whether due to illness, accident or aging, can lead to significant respiratory complications. Indeed, immobility or reduced physical activity directly affects the respiratory system by limiting pulmonary expansion, promoting the accumulation of bronchial secretions, and increasing the risk of complications such as lung infections. Understanding this interrelationship enables us to adapt care and prevent respiratory complications in people with reduced mobility.

# 1. Reduced mobility and its impact on respiratory mechanics

Movement is essential for maintaining optimal respiratory function. **Mobility** enables the lungs to expand and contract correctly, promoting efficient **gas exchange**. When mobility is reduced, respiratory mechanics are compromised, leading to a series of adverse consequences for breathing.

## Decreased thoracic expansion

In a healthy, mobile person, the diaphragm and intercostal muscles ensure good **lung expansion** during inspiration. However, when a person is immobile or bedridden for long periods, ribcage expansion is limited, reducing **total lung capacity**.

- **Poor use of the diaphragm**: The **diaphragm**, the main respiratory muscle, needs movement to contract and allow full inspiration. When the person remains motionless, the diaphragm can contract less efficiently, resulting in **shallow inspirations** and **inefficient ventilation**. This limits the amount of air entering the lungs, reducing gas exchange.

- **Reduced lung volumes**: Prolonged immobility leads to a reduction in **lung volumes such as** tidal volume (the amount of air inhaled and exhaled during each respiratory cycle) and vital capacity. This reduction limits oxygen intake and promotes **carbon dioxide retention**, particularly in patients with respiratory diseases such as COPD.

## Weakness of respiratory muscles

**Muscle weakness** linked to immobility affects not only the muscles of the limbs and trunk, but also the **respiratory muscles**, such as the diaphragm, intercostal and abdominal muscles. This makes breathing less efficient.

- **Atrophy of respiratory muscles**: In the absence of movement and regular physical activity, respiratory muscles can atrophy. This reduces their capacity to generate the force required for complete inspiration and expiration, leading to **shallow breathing** and alveolar **hypoventilation** (insufficient ventilation of the alveoli).

240

- **Decreased coughing strength**: Coughing is an essential mechanism for **expelling** accumulated **secretions from** the respiratory tract. In the event of muscular weakness, **coughing force** is reduced, making it more difficult to eliminate mucus and promoting the accumulation of secretions, thus increasing the risk of pulmonary infection and airway obstruction.

## 2. Accumulation of secretions and risk of pulmonary infections

One of the main side-effects of reduced mobility on breathing is the **accumulation of bronchial secretions**. In the supine position or during prolonged immobility, it becomes difficult to **mobilize secretions**, and people who are bedridden or not very active are often unable to expectorate them properly. This accumulation of mucus creates an environment conducive to infection.

### Difficulty draining secretions

When people move less, the **natural drainage of secretions** in the respiratory tract is compromised. Normally, body movement helps to dislodge and circulate mucus from the bronchial tubes to the trachea, where it can be eliminated by coughing.

- **Mucus stagnation**: In people with reduced mobility, bronchial secretions stagnate in the lower airways, increasing the risk of obstruction and **alveolar collapse** (atelectasis), a condition in which part of the lung collapses, reducing the surface area available for gas exchange.

### Increased risk of lung infections

Immobility associated with an accumulation of secretions also favours the development of **pulmonary infections**, such as pneumonia. Bacteria and viruses can proliferate in retained

241

secretions, leading to serious infections, particularly in the elderly or immunocompromised.

- **Hypostatic pneumonia**: This type of pneumonia develops in people confined to bed for long periods, due to **stagnation of secretions** in the lower parts of the lungs. This phenomenon is common in hospitalized patients or those recovering from surgery.

- **Exacerbation of respiratory diseases**: in patients with **COPD** or **asthma**, immobility can worsen **secretion retention** and promote **exacerbations of** the disease, increasing symptoms such as dyspnea, coughing and chest tightness.

## 3. Impact of body position on breathing

**Body position** has a significant impact on respiratory function. People with reduced mobility or who are immobilized often have to remain in a sitting or lying position for long periods, which further compromises their breathing.

### Lying down and its negative effects

When patients **lie on their backs** for long periods, **gravity** exerts pressure on the lungs and other thoracic organs, limiting their expansion. This reduces lung capacity, especially in the **lung bases**, which are essential for oxygenation.

- **Lung compression**: in the supine position, the **abdominal organs** exert pressure on the diaphragm, reducing its excursion and thus the lungs' capacity to fill with air. This hypoventilates the lower lobes of the lungs, encouraging secretions to accumulate in these areas.

- **Hypoxia**: Lack of adequate ventilation of the lung bases can lead to **hypoxia** (reduced oxygen levels in the blood), especially in patients with chronic lung disease.

Insufficient oxygenation of vital organs aggravates fatigue and physical deconditioning.

**Advantages of the semi-seated or Fowler position**

To improve breathing in immobile people, the **semi-seated** (or **Fowler) position**, where the patient is reclined at an angle of 30 to 45 degrees, is often recommended.

- **Improved lung expansion**: the semi-seated position enables **better thoracic expansion by** releasing the pressure exerted by the abdominal organs on the diaphragm. This facilitates breathing and improves gas exchange.

- **Preventing secretion build-up**: By being slightly upright, the person can better **clear the respiratory tract** and facilitate mucus evacuation by coughing or postural drainage. This position is particularly useful for the elderly or patients with chronic lung conditions.

## 4. Early mobilization and respiratory rehabilitation

To prevent respiratory complications associated with reduced mobility, **early mobilization** and **respiratory rehabilitation** are crucial. These interventions help improve lung function, stimulate circulation and reduce the risk of infection.

**Early mobilization after surgery or in hospital**

In hospitalized patients, it is essential to promote **early mobilization** as soon as their condition allows. This may involve **light** sitting **exercises**, walking aids, or passive breathing exercises.

- **Breathing exercises**: Patients can be encouraged to practice **deep breathing** exercises, focusing on diaphragmatic breathing to improve lung expansion and reduce secretion build-up.

- **Mobility aid**: Even limited movement, such as walking around the room or getting out of bed, helps **ventilation** and reduces the risk of **atelectasis** or pneumonia.

**Respiratory rehabilitation and physical therapy**

**Respiratory rehabilitation** plays a crucial role for people suffering from chronic respiratory diseases or physical deconditioning due to prolonged immobility.

- **Bronchial drainage techniques**: **Respiratory physiotherapy** helps to mobilize accumulated secretions and clear the airways. Techniques such as **chest percussion**, **vibration** or **controlled coughing exercises** are frequently used to promote expectoration.

- **Muscle-strengthening exercises**: Respiratory rehabilitation also includes exercises to strengthen the respiratory muscles. These exercises, often performed in conjunction with a physiotherapist, are designed to improve the ability to inhale deeply and expel air efficiently from the lungs.

- **Managing multiple medications in elderly respiratory patients**
  ○ Drug interactions related to respiratory diseases

**Drug interactions** linked to **respiratory pathologies** represent a crucial issue in the management of patients, particularly those suffering from chronic diseases such as **chronic obstructive pulmonary disease (COPD), asthma** or **respiratory insufficiency**. Indeed, people suffering from these conditions are often poly-medicated, due to the management of their underlying disease, but also frequent co-morbidities (such as hypertension, diabetes or cardiovascular disorders). This multiple use of treatments can expose patients to potential **drug interactions** that influence the efficacy of respiratory treatments, or even cause serious adverse reactions.

# 1. Bronchodilators and their interactions

**Bronchodilators** are essential medications in the management of chronic respiratory diseases such as **COPD** and **asthma**. They work by relaxing airway muscles to facilitate breathing. However, these drugs can interact with other treatments, which can compromise their efficacy or cause adverse effects.

### Interactions with beta-agonists

**Beta-2** agonists (such as **salbutamol, formoterol** or **terbutaline**) are frequently used as inhalers to treat COPD and asthma. These drugs can cause systemic effects by stimulating beta receptors in other organs, notably the heart.

- **Interactions with beta-blockers** : Patients with respiratory diseases may also be treated for cardiovascular disorders with **beta-blockers** (drugs used to treat hypertension or heart rhythm disorders). However, beta-agonists, especially **non-selective** ones (such as **propranolol**), can **antagonize the effects of beta-agonists**, reducing their bronchodilator efficacy and exacerbating respiratory symptoms. They may also increase the risk of bronchospasm in asthmatic patients.

- **Interactions with diuretics**: Beta-2 agonists can cause **hypokalemia** (reduced potassium levels in the blood), an effect which may be exacerbated by the concomitant use of **thiazide diuretics** or **loop diuretics** (such as **furosemide**). Severe hypokalemia may lead to cardiac rhythm disturbances and require increased electrolyte monitoring.

### Interactions with anticholinergics

**Anticholinergics** such as **tiotropium** and **ipratropium** are also commonly used bronchodilators in the management of chronic respiratory pathologies, notably COPD.

- **Interactions with other anticholinergics**: Concomitant use of other anticholinergic drugs (such as certain **tricyclic antidepressants, antihistamines** or **antiparkinsonian agents**) may cause adverse effects associated with anticholinergic overload. These include **dry mouth, blurred vision, urinary retention**, and in extreme cases, cognitive impairment and confusion in the elderly.

- **Interactions with Parkinson's disease drugs**: In patients with Parkinson's disease, anticholinergic therapies used for COPD may **interact** with antiparkinsonian drugs (such as **levodopa**), exacerbating neurological side effects or compromising the efficacy of both treatments.

## 2. Inhaled and systemic corticosteroids

**Corticosteroids** are widely used for their anti-inflammatory effect in the management of chronic respiratory diseases, whether in inhaled or systemic (oral or intravenous) form. Although effective, corticosteroids can lead to significant **drug interactions**, especially when used on a long-term basis.

### Interactions with antidiabetic drugs

**Systemic** corticosteroids (such as **prednisone**) can cause **hyperglycemia** by increasing insulin resistance. In diabetic patients, this can make glycemic control more difficult.

- **Reduced efficacy of antidiabetic agents**: Corticosteroid-induced hyperglycemia may necessitate **adaptation of antidiabetic therapy**, particularly in patients on **insulin**

246

or **oral antidiabetic agents** (such as **metformin** or **hypoglycemic sulfonamides**). Regular blood glucose monitoring is essential to prevent diabetic complications.

**Interactions with anticoagulants**

Systemic corticosteroids can also interact with **anticoagulants** (such as **warfarin**). This interaction can be complex, as corticosteroids can **alter the metabolism of anticoagulants**, leading either to an increased risk of bleeding (through anticoagulant overdosage), or to a reduction in their efficacy.

- **Increased monitoring**: in patients taking both corticosteroids and anticoagulants, regular monitoring of **INR** (International Normalized Ratio) **levels** is essential to adjust doses and avoid clotting complications.

**Interactions with immunosuppressive drugs**

Long-term use of corticosteroids, particularly in high doses, can lead to **immunosuppression**. This increases the risk of opportunistic infections, particularly in patients also taking other **immunosuppressants** (such as those used after organ transplants or to treat autoimmune diseases). It is essential to closely monitor the immune status of patients on combination therapy.

# 3. Antibiotics and antifungals for respiratory infections

**Antibiotics** and **antifungals** are frequently prescribed for patients with respiratory diseases, particularly pneumonia, bronchopulmonary infections and superinfections in COPD. However, some of these drugs may interact with background treatments for respiratory diseases, or even with each other.

**Interactions with macrolides**

**Macrolides** (such as **azithromycin** or **clarithromycin**) are antibiotics commonly used to treat respiratory infections. However, they can cause significant drug interactions.

- **Interactions with bronchodilators**: Macrolides can increase plasma concentrations of certain bronchodilators, by inhibiting cytochrome P450 enzymes (notably CYP3A4). For example, they can increase levels of **theophylline**, a bronchodilator still sometimes used, thereby increasing the risk of **toxicity** (nausea, vomiting, arrhythmias).

- **Interactions with anticoagulants** : Macrolides can also **prolong the effect of anticoagulants such as** warfarin, increasing the risk of bleeding. In patients on anticoagulants, INR monitoring is essential when prescribing macrolides.

**Interactions with antifungal agents**

**Azole antifungals** (such as **fluconazole** or **itraconazole**) are used to treat respiratory fungal infections, which can occur in immunocompromised patients or those on corticosteroid therapy. These drugs also inhibit **cytochrome P450**, which can lead to serious interactions.

- **Increased corticosteroid concentrations**: Azole antifungals can increase plasma concentrations of **inhaled** or systemic **corticosteroids**, by slowing down their metabolism. This can lead to **systemic** corticosteroid **side effects**, such as hyperglycemia, hypertension, or even **Cushing's syndrome** (weight gain, round face, muscle weakness).

# 4. Interactions with other common treatments

Patients with respiratory pathologies, particularly the elderly, often have **co-morbidities** (diabetes, hypertension, cardiovascular disorders) requiring additional treatments. These drugs can sometimes interact with respiratory treatments.

**Interactions with antihypertensives**

**Antihypertensives**, such as angiotensin-converting enzyme (ACE) inhibitors or angiotensin II receptor blockers (ARB-II), are often prescribed for patients with chronic respiratory disease, due to the frequent association between hypertension and COPD.

- **ACE-induced cough: ACE inhibitors** (such as **ramipril** or **enalapril**) can cause **dry cough** in some patients, a side effect that can be confused with respiratory symptoms. This can complicate the management of chronic respiratory disease and necessitate a change in antihypertensive treatment to an ARB-II (such as **losartan**), which does not cause this side effect.

**Interactions with sedatives and opioids**

**Sedatives, hypnotics** and **opioids** are sometimes used to treat anxiety, insomnia or pain in patients with respiratory pathologies. However, these drugs can **depress the respiratory system**, increasing the risk of respiratory failure.

- **Respiratory depression**: Opioids (such as **morphine** or **fentanyl**) and benzodiazepines (such as **diazepam**) can cause **respiratory depression** by reducing the sensitivity of the brain's respiratory centers to carbon dioxide. This interaction is particularly dangerous in patients with severe COPD or chronic respiratory insufficiency.

**Monitoring treatment efficacy** and **managing side effects** are crucial steps in the management of patients with respiratory pathologies, particularly those suffering from chronic diseases such as **asthma, chronic obstructive pulmonary disease (COPD)** or **respiratory failure**. These patients require long-term treatments that need to be regularly re-evaluated to ensure they are achieving their therapeutic objectives, while minimizing **adverse effects**. Proactive monitoring not only makes it possible to adjust doses or drug combinations, but also to maintain patients' quality of life by avoiding complications.

# 1. Monitoring treatment efficacy

The first step in the management of respiratory diseases is to check whether prescribed treatments are achieving the desired results, i.e. improvement in symptoms and lung function. This monitoring is based both on **objective** examinations and on the **evaluation of symptoms** reported by the patient.

**Monitoring clinical symptoms**

One of the main ways to assess the effectiveness of a treatment is to monitor the patient's **respiratory symptoms**, including **dyspnea** (shortness of breath), **cough, wheezing** and **sputum**.

- **Asthma**: In an asthmatic patient, the effectiveness of treatment is measured by the **reduction in the frequency** and **severity of asthma attacks**, and the ability to prevent exacerbations. The patient must also be able to resume normal physical activities without excessive respiratory discomfort.

- **COPD**: For COPD patients, the efficacy of treatment is assessed by an improvement in **exercise tolerance**, a **reduction in** day-to-day **dyspnea**, and a **reduction in exacerbations**. If symptoms persist or worsen despite

250

regular treatment, this may indicate the need to adjust dosage or consider a different background therapy.

- **Respiratory failure**: In cases of chronic respiratory failure, the aim of treatment is to maintain **adequate oxygenation**. Effectiveness is measured by the reduction of hypoxia-related symptoms, such as **fatigue, cyanosis** or cognitive impairment. A patient well stabilized on oxygen therapy or non-invasive ventilation (NIV) should show a marked improvement in respiratory function.

**Objective measurements of lung function**

To more accurately assess the effectiveness of respiratory treatments, **pulmonary function tests** are carried out on a regular basis. They provide objective data for fine-tuning treatments.

- **Spirometry**: Spirometry is one of the most widely used tests for monitoring patients with asthma or COPD. It measures **lung capacity** and respiratory flow (FEV1, FVC). A stable or improving FEV1 (forced expiratory volume in one second) suggests that treatment is effective. On the other hand, a deterioration in results may indicate disease progression or a need for therapeutic modification.

- **Blood gases**: In patients with respiratory failure, **arterial blood gases** are used to measure **oxygen ($PaO_2$)** and **carbon dioxide ($PaCO_2$)** levels in the blood. An improvement in $PaO_2$ values and stabilization of $PaCO_2$ indicate that oxygen therapy or ventilation treatment is effective. A deterioration in blood gases may necessitate adjustment of oxygen therapy or the introduction of assisted ventilation.

- **Pulse oximetry**: In ambulatory care, **pulse oximetry** is a non-invasive method of monitoring oxygen saturation ($SpO_2$). An $SpO_2$ between 92 and 96% in a patient with COPD or respiratory failure is generally considered

251

satisfactory. Recurrent falls in SpO2 below 88% call for a reassessment of treatment.

## 2. Managing the side effects of respiratory treatments

While treatments are effective in controlling symptoms, they can sometimes lead to **side effects that** affect the patient's quality of life. Proactive management of these side effects is therefore essential to ensure adherence to treatment and prevent serious complications.

**Side effects of bronchodilators**

**Bronchodilators**, whether **beta-2** agonists (salbutamol, formoterol) or **anticholinergics** (ipratropium, tiotropium), are essential for the management of asthma and COPD, but they can cause side effects, particularly when used in high doses.

- **Tachycardia and palpitations**: Beta-2 agonists can cause excessive **cardiac stimulation**, leading to palpitations or tachycardia. These symptoms should be monitored, particularly in patients with a history of heart disease. If these effects are too troublesome, dose adjustment or a change of medication may be necessary.

- **Dry mouth**: Anticholinergics such as tiotropium can cause **significant dry mouth**, making treatment unpleasant. It is important to advise the patient to take simple measures, such as drinking small amounts of water frequently or using a moisturizing mouth spray.

- **Muscle cramps and tremors**: Beta-2 agonists can also cause **muscle tremors** or **cramps**. These effects are generally dose-dependent and can be reduced by adjusting the drug's dosage.

## Side effects of corticosteroids

**Corticosteroids**, whether inhaled or systemic, play a key role in reducing airway inflammation. However, they are also associated with a range of side effects, particularly when used over long periods.

- **Oral candidiasis (thrush): Inhaled corticosteroids**, such as budesonide or fluticasone, can cause a **fungal infection** of the mouth and throat, known as oral candidiasis. To prevent this, patients are advised to rinse their mouths after each inhalation. In the event of recurrent candidiasis, a consultation is necessary to adjust treatment.

- **Skin fragility and osteoporosis: Systemic corticosteroids**, especially when taken long-term, can cause systemic side effects such as **skin fragility**, **osteoporosis** and weight gain. In patients on long-term corticosteroid therapy, it is essential to monitor **bone density** and prescribe **calcium and vitamin D supplements** to prevent bone loss.

- **Risk of infection**: Corticosteroids reduce the activity of the immune system, thus increasing the risk of **infections**. Close monitoring is necessary, especially for signs of pulmonary infection, and vaccinations (e.g. against influenza and pneumococcus) must be kept up to date.

## Side effects of antibiotics and other treatments

Patients suffering from chronic respiratory diseases, particularly COPD, are often prone to frequent infections requiring **antibiotics**. While these treatments are essential, they can also have undesirable effects that need to be monitored.

- **Gastrointestinal disorders**: Antibiotics, particularly macrolides (azithromycin), can cause **digestive disorders** such as diarrhea or nausea. In sensitive patients, it may be necessary to recommend **probiotics** to prevent imbalances in intestinal flora.

- **Risk of resistance**: Prolonged use of antibiotics is associated with an increased risk of **bacterial resistance**. It is therefore essential to use antibiotics only when necessary, and to strictly adhere to dosage and duration of treatment to avoid the emergence of resistant strains.

## 3. Treatment adaptation and long-term follow-up

The management of patients with chronic respiratory pathologies is dynamic, requiring **regular adaptation of treatments** according to the patient's response, the appearance of side effects and the evolution of the disease.

### Dosage adjustment

If a treatment is ineffective or poorly tolerated, it may be necessary to adjust dosage or change medication. Patients should be closely monitored during any change to ensure that there is no clinical deterioration or new adverse effects.

- **Reassessment of bronchodilators**: in COPD patients, it's common to adjust the dose of bronchodilators or combine several (beta-agonist and anticholinergic) to improve efficacy while limiting side effects.

- **Corticosteroid titration**: Corticosteroids should be used at the minimum effective dose to limit long-term adverse effects. If symptoms are well controlled, a gradual reduction in dose may be considered.

### Regular follow-up and patient education

Regular patient follow-up is essential to assess treatment efficacy and the impact of side effects. Appropriate education of patients about their disease and treatment is also crucial to ensure long-term adherence.

- **Therapeutic education**: Patients need to be informed about the objectives of their treatment, the signs indicating an exacerbation of their disease, and the potential side effects to watch out for. A well-informed patient is more likely to report problems promptly and adhere to treatment.

- **Long-term follow-up**: Regular consultations, lung function tests and symptom evaluation enable us to monitor disease progression and adjust treatments according to the patient's changing needs.

# Chapter 10

# Prevention of nosocomial infections in pneumology

- **Common nosocomial infections in pneumology**
  - ○ Ventilator-associated pneumonia, respiratory tract infections

**Ventilator-associated pneumonia** (VAP) and **respiratory tract infections** are frequent and serious complications in mechanically ventilated patients. They occur in the hospital setting, mainly in intensive care units, and are associated with **high mortality**, **longer hospital stays** and **increased healthcare costs**. Mechanical ventilation, while essential to maintain oxygenation and support breathing in patients in respiratory distress, is a major risk factor for respiratory infections. Good care management, combined with rigorous prevention, is essential to limit these complications.

# 1. Understanding ventilation-associated pneumonia

**Ventilator-associated pneumonia (VAP(** is defined as a pulmonary infection that occurs at least **48 to 72 hours** after a patient has been intubated. The risk of developing VAP increases with the duration of mechanical ventilator use. Ventilation promotes colonization of the lower respiratory tract by pathogenic bacteria and compromises natural defense mechanisms, making patients vulnerable to infection.

**Mechanisms of VAP**

The **pathophysiological mechanisms** responsible for ventilation-associated pneumonia involve several factors. Mechanically ventilated patients are unable to effectively clear bronchial secretions, and tracheal intubation creates a **direct portal of entry for pathogens** into the lower respiratory tract.

- **Aspiration of oropharyngeal secretions**: Intubation disrupts the respiratory tract's natural defenses, notably the closure of the larynx, and favors the **aspiration of** oropharyngeal secretions containing bacteria. This is particularly true for patients in supine position or with gastro-oesophageal reflux disease.

258

- **Colonization of medical devices**: Endotracheal tubes and ventilation circuits can be **colonized by bacteria**, creating a reservoir for the proliferation of pathogens. Bacteria sometimes form biofilms on these devices, making them difficult to eradicate and increasing the risk of pulmonary infection.

- **Retention of bronchial secretions**: The reduced ability to **expectorate secretions** increases the risk of mucus accumulation in the respiratory tract. This stagnation provides an environment conducive to the proliferation of pathogens, promoting infection.

**Pathogens involved in VAP**

The pathogens responsible for ventilator-associated pneumonia are generally **bacteria** and, more rarely, **fungi** or **viruses**. The bacteria involved are often nosocomial germs, difficult to treat because of their **resistance to antibiotics**.

- **Gram-negative bacteria**: **Enterobacteriaceae** such as *Klebsiella pneumoniae*, *Escherichia coli* and *Pseudomonas aeruginosa* are frequently isolated from patients suffering from VAP. These bacteria are often resistant to several classes of antibiotics, which complicates their management.

- **Methicillin-resistant Staphylococcus aureus (MRSA)**: This Gram-positive bacterium is a frequent cause of VAP, particularly in long-term hospitalized patients or those who have been exposed to multiple courses of antibiotics.

- **Opportunistic pathogens**: Patients who are immunocompromised or on prolonged corticosteroid therapy are also at risk of infection from fungi such as *Candida* and *Aspergillus*, or viruses such as **herpesvirus** or **cytomegalovirus**.

## 2. Risk factors for ventilator-associated pneumonia

Certain risk factors increase the likelihood of developing ventilator-associated pneumonia, including the duration of mechanical ventilation and the patient's general condition.

### Duration of mechanical ventilation

The **main risk factor** for VAP is the **duration of exposure to mechanical ventilation**. The longer a patient is ventilated, the greater the risk of pulmonary infection. It has been estimated that each additional day on mechanical ventilation increases the risk of VAP by **1-3%**.

### Immune status and comorbidities

Patients with **co-morbidities** (such as COPD, heart failure or diabetes) or those who are **immunocompromised** are more likely to develop serious ventilator-associated infections. In addition, immunosuppressive treatments such as **corticosteroids** also increase vulnerability to nosocomial infections.

### Nutrition and deconditioning

**Malnutrition** is another important risk factor. Malnourished patients have a reduced capacity to fight infection, due to a weakened immune system. In addition, prolonged immobility, common in ventilated patients, contributes to **physical deconditioning**, which exacerbates the risk of infectious complications.

## 3. Diagnosis of ventilation-associated pneumonia

The diagnosis of ventilation-associated pneumonia is based on a combination of **clinical signs**, **biological parameters** and

**radiological findings**. Diagnosis can be difficult, as classic signs of pneumonia, such as fever and productive cough, may be masked in patients under sedation and mechanical ventilation.

### Clinical signs

The main clinical signs that may suggest pneumonia in a ventilated patient are :

- Persistent **fever** or further rise in temperature.
- **Hypoxemia**: A drop in oxygen saturation (SpO2) despite assisted ventilation.
- **Purulent sputum** in bronchial secretions.
- **Hemodynamic alterations**: unexplained hypotension or tachycardia may also be a sign of pulmonary infection.

### Imaging and microbiological sampling

- **Chest X-ray**: A newly appearing **pulmonary infiltration** on a chest X-ray is a suggestive sign of VAP. However, it can be difficult to distinguish infections from other causes of lung damage, such as pulmonary edema or atelectasis.

- **Microbiological sampling**: Microbiological confirmation is achieved by **bronchial sampling** (tracheal or bronchoalveolar aspiration), followed by bacterial culture. This helps identify the germs responsible and guide antibiotic treatment.

## 4. Treatment of ventilation-associated pneumonia

Treatment of VAP relies primarily on the administration of **broad-spectrum antibiotics,** tailored to the germs identified by microbiological sampling. Treatment must be initiated rapidly to prevent infection progression and serious complications.

**Antibiotic therapy**

- **Empirical antibiotic therapy**: While awaiting culture results, **empirical antibiotic therapy** is usually started, based on local protocols and knowledge of the most likely nosocomial germs in each facility. This often includes antibiotics covering both **Gram-negative** and **methicillin-resistant Staphylococcus aureus**.

- **De-escalation**: Once culture results are available, antibiotic therapy is **readjusted** according to the germs isolated and their sensitivity. This approach, known as **de-escalation**, limits the use of broad-spectrum antibiotics and reduces the risk of developing bacterial resistance.

**Support measures**

In addition to antibiotic therapy, **supportive measures** are essential to improve the patient's clinical condition. These include:

- **Oxygen therapy** or adjustment of ventilation to maintain adequate oxygen saturation.
- **Postural drainage** and **respiratory physiotherapy** to help evacuate bronchial secretions and improve ventilation.

## 5. Prevention of ventilation-associated pneumonia

**Preventing** VAP is essential, as it is one of the most feared nosocomial infections in intensive care. Several preventive strategies have been shown to be effective in reducing the incidence of these infections.

**Hygiene and asepsis**

- **Hand hygiene**: Caregivers must **disinfect their hands** before and after handling the ventilator or patient, to prevent the transmission of bacteria.

- **Maintenance of medical devices**: The ventilation circuit must be changed regularly, and care of the intubation site must be carried out under **strict aseptic** conditions to avoid bacterial colonization.

**Positional precautions**

Patient position plays a key role in preventing VAP. It is recommended to keep the patient in a **semi-seated** position (30-45 degree angle) to reduce the risk of **aspiration of** oropharyngeal **secretions** into the lungs.

**Use of minimal sedation**

**Minimal sedation** and **early extubation** are also essential. Reducing the duration of mechanical ventilation significantly reduces the risk of VAP. As soon as the patient's clinical condition allows, an attempt is made to wean the patient off the ventilator.

  ◦    The role of hygiene and sanitary protocols

**Hygiene and sanitary protocols** play a fundamental **role** in infection prevention, particularly in healthcare environments where patients are often vulnerable due to their state of health. These measures are essential to protect patients, caregivers and all hospital staff from nosocomial infections (hospital-acquired infections), such as pneumonia, urinary tract infections and septicemia. Rigorous application of **hygiene protocols** and **sanitary practices** reduces the spread of pathogens and significantly improves the quality of care.

263

# 1. Importance of hygiene in care environments

Hygiene in healthcare facilities goes far beyond conventional cleaning. It encompasses a set of practices designed to **prevent the transmission of infectious agents**, such as bacteria, viruses and fungi, which can circulate between patients, caregivers and medical devices. The reduction of **nosocomial infections** depends to a large extent on compliance with health protocols in all phases of medical care.

### Hand hygiene: the first line of defense

Hand washing is the **basic** and most effective **measure** for preventing the transmission of infections in hospitals and other healthcare facilities. **Hand-to-hand transmission**, i.e. the transmission of germs via the hands, is one of the main vectors of contamination.

- **Simple washing and disinfection**: It's essential that nursing staff, doctors and even visitors wash their hands with soap or disinfect them with hydroalcoholic solutions before and after any contact with a patient or medical equipment. These practices considerably reduce the microbial load.

- **Critical moments for hand hygiene**: The World Health Organization (WHO) has defined five key moments for hand hygiene, notably before touching a patient, after contact with body fluids, or after handling potentially contaminated equipment.

### Hygiene of medical devices

Medical devices such as **catheters, endotracheal tubes** and **ventilators** are potential sources of infection if not properly cleaned and disinfected. Compliance with **sterilization** and

**disinfection** protocols is essential to prevent colonization of equipment by pathogens.

- **Regular disinfection**: Reusable medical devices, such as endoscopes or ventilation equipment, must be thoroughly disinfected between uses to prevent cross-transmission between patients. Similarly, surfaces around patients must be cleaned regularly to prevent contamination.

- **Waste and fluid management**: The correct handling of medical waste, such as soiled bandages or used syringes, and the safe management of body fluids, are crucial to preventing infection. These products must be disposed of safely in accordance with current protocols.

## 2. Health protocols for infection prevention

**Health protocols** are sets of rules and practices designed to standardize hygiene and prevention measures in healthcare environments. Their aim is to reduce the risk of contamination and infection for patients and healthcare staff. These protocols are often based on international guidelines, such as those issued by the WHO or the Centers for Disease Control and Prevention (CDC).

### Standard and additional precautions

**Standard precautions** apply to all patients, whatever their infectious status, and are implemented to prevent the transmission of micro-organisms via blood, secretions or excretions.

- **Personal protective equipment (PPE)**: Wearing protective equipment, such as **gloves**, **masks** and **gowns**, is part of the basic measures to protect caregivers and patients from pathogens. **Masks** are essential to prevent the transmission of respiratory infections, especially in the case of droplet-borne diseases such as tuberculosis or influenza.

- **Additional precautions**: In addition to standard precautions, specific precautions may be required for certain patients with highly contagious or treatment-resistant infections, such as **methicillin-resistant Staphylococcus aureus (MRSA)**. These precautions include patient isolation, the use of patient-specific equipment and reinforced disinfection measures.

## Asepsis protocols for invasive procedures

**Invasive procedures** such as catheter placement, intubation or surgery are high-risk situations for the introduction of infections. **Surgical asepsis** protocols aim to ensure that these procedures are carried out under sterile conditions to avoid contamination.

- **Instrument sterilization** : Instruments used during an invasive procedure must be **sterile** and handled according to strict aseptic techniques to prevent the introduction of germs into the patient's body.

- **Skin antisepsis**: Before any surgical procedure or the insertion of an invasive device, the patient's skin is disinfected with an **antiseptic**, such as chlorhexidine or betadine, to eliminate bacteria present on the skin surface and reduce the risk of infection.

## Ventilation and air control

**Air quality** control is an essential element in preventing infections, particularly respiratory infections. Ventilation systems, particularly in operating theatres and intensive care units, must be designed to limit the circulation of organisms-micro in the air.

- **Negative and positive pressure**: In some wards, such as isolation rooms, a **negative pressure** system is used to prevent germs present in the room from spreading to other parts of the hospital. Conversely, operating theatres use

**positive pressure systems** to prevent the entry of outside germs.

- **Air filtration**: **HEPA** (High-Efficiency Particulate Air) **filtration** systems are used in sensitive environments, such as intensive care units, to filter out fine particles and prevent the spread of airborne pathogens.

# 3. Impact of health protocols on nosocomial infections

**Nosocomial infections**, which occur in patients hospitalized for another reason, are a major threat in hospitals and care facilities. They are responsible for increased morbidity and mortality, as well as higher hospital costs. Strict application of health protocols can significantly reduce their incidence.

### Reduced respiratory infections

**Respiratory infections**, such as **ventilator-associated pneumonia**, are among the most frequent and serious nosocomial infections. These infections occur mainly in mechanically ventilated patients, often as a result of bacterial colonization of the airways.

- **Pneumonia prevention**: Specific protocols for ventilated patients, such as maintaining the **semi-seated position** (Fowler), using single-use or rigorously disinfected ventilation devices, and regular mouth care, significantly reduce the risk of ventilation-associated pneumonia.

### Prevention of urinary tract infections and sepsis

Urinary tract infections, often caused by prolonged catheter placement, and septicemia are also common nosocomial infections. To prevent these infections, it is essential to comply with protocols for managing medical devices and preventing contamination.

- **Catheter management**: **Urinary catheters** must be inserted and maintained in accordance with strict aseptic rules. They should be removed as soon as they are no longer required, to limit the risk of infection.

- **Monitoring for signs of infection**: Caregivers need to be trained to recognize **early signs of infection** in patients, so they can respond quickly with appropriate treatment. This includes monitoring vital parameters, body temperature and laboratory results.

## 4. Education and training of nursing staff

To ensure that **hygiene and sanitation protocols** are consistently observed, it is vital that care staff receive **ongoing training** and are regularly made aware of the importance of these measures. Awareness-raising campaigns on hand hygiene, reminders of asepsis precautions and training in the use of personal protective equipment (PPE) are essential to ensure safe care.

- **Simulations and workshops**: Organizing **simulations** and **practical workshops** on medical device management and hygiene procedures helps to reinforce the skills of care staff. Regular exercises help maintain a high level of vigilance.

- **Regular audits and controls**: To ensure that protocols are respected at all times, **regular** internal **audits** can be set up. These audits enable us to assess practices, detect any shortcomings in the application of protocols and take any necessary corrective action.

- **Disinfection protocol for respiratory devices**
  - Maintenance of oxygen therapy and assisted ventilation equipment

The **maintenance of oxygen therapy and assisted ventilation equipment** is fundamental to the effective management of patients requiring respiratory assistance. This equipment is used both in hospital and at home, often for prolonged periods. Rigorous maintenance and appropriate disinfection protocols are essential to avoid technical malfunctions and, above all, to prevent respiratory infections linked to the use of medical devices. The aim is to ensure that oxygen therapy and assisted ventilation equipment, such as **oxygen spectacles, masks** or **mechanical ventilators**, are not only efficient, but also safe for the patient.

# 1. Importance of regular maintenance

Oxygen therapy and assisted ventilation equipment are in direct contact with the patient's respiratory tract, a sensitive environment for contamination. If equipment is not properly maintained, it can become a reservoir for germs, increasing the risk of **respiratory infections** such as pneumonia. What's more, poorly maintained equipment can develop **technical faults**, reducing the effectiveness of care or leading to serious complications for the patient.

**Preventing nosocomial infections**

Infections associated with the use of respiratory equipment are mainly due to **microbial colonization of** the devices (oxygen goggles, masks, filters, tubing). Bacteria, especially hospital pathogens such as *Pseudomonas aeruginosa* or *Staphylococcus aureus*, can proliferate on moist respiratory equipment.

- **Regular cleaning and disinfection**: Regular cleaning of equipment with appropriate disinfectant solutions eliminates bacteria and organic deposits (mucus, saliva).

Rigorous disinfection must be carried out after each use in hospital wards, or according to a strict schedule at home.

- **Replacing single-use components**: Single-use components, such as filters and tubing, should be replaced after each use or at regular intervals, as recommended by the manufacturer. This minimizes the risk of infection.

### Maintaining device performance

Another key aspect of equipment maintenance is to ensure that oxygen therapy and assisted ventilation devices function correctly to meet the patient's respiratory needs.

- **Checking oxygen flow rates**: For oxygen therapy systems such as **oxygen concentrators or compressed oxygen cylinders**, it is essential to ensure that oxygen flow rates are correctly set and consistently delivered. An undetected drop in flow can lead to hypoxia, while too high a flow can cause hyperoxia, which is harmful in the long term.

- **Assessment of ventilation systems**: In the case of assisted ventilation (CPAP, BiPAP, mechanical ventilators), maintenance aims to check the quality of **ventilation delivered**, as well as the correct operation of safety alarms and pressure systems. Poorly adjusted equipment can cause under-ventilation or barotrauma, particularly dangerous for patients with severe respiratory pathologies.

## 2. Maintenance of oxygen therapy devices

**Oxygen therapy** is commonly used for patients suffering from **chronic respiratory diseases** such as **COPD, respiratory failure** or **acute asthma exacerbations**. It can be administered **via oxygen goggles, masks** or **oxygen tents**. Each of these devices requires specific maintenance.

## Oxygen goggles and masks

**Nasal cannula** and **oxygen masks** are the most commonly used interfaces for oxygen administration. Their maintenance is designed to prevent secretion build-up and microbial contamination.

- **Daily cleaning**: Oxygen goggles and masks should be cleaned daily with lukewarm water and mild soap, then rinsed thoroughly with clear water to remove any soap residue, which could irritate the respiratory tract. Homecare patients must be trained to perform this task independently or with the help of caregivers.

- **Regular replacement**: Even with careful maintenance, oxygen masks and goggles deteriorate over time. They must be replaced regularly to ensure a good seal and avoid any risk of oxygen leakage or loss of efficiency.

## Tubes and humidifiers

Particular attention must also be paid to the **tubing** connecting oxygen therapy devices to oxygen concentrators or oxygen cylinders.

- **Checking tubing**: Tubing should be regularly inspected for **cracks** or **kinks**, which could compromise correct oxygen delivery. Damaged tubing should be replaced immediately.

- **Humidifier maintenance**: Oxygen can dry out respiratory mucous membranes, so **humidifiers** are often used to moisten inspired air. However, these devices can become reservoirs for bacteria if the water is not changed regularly. Distilled water should be used, and humidifiers should be cleaned and disinfected at least once a day.

# 3. Maintenance of assisted ventilation systems

**Assisted ventilation** devices (such as **non-invasive ventilation** via **CPAP** or **BiPAP**, as well as mechanical ventilators) are used for patients suffering from acute or chronic respiratory failure. These systems are particularly complex, and require regular, rigorous maintenance to ensure their smooth operation.

**Non-invasive ventilation: CPAP and BiPAP**

**CPAP** (continuous positive airway pressure) and **BiPAP** (bi-level positive airway pressure) machines are used to keep the airways open, particularly in patients suffering from **sleep apnea** or **COPD**. Their maintenance is crucial to avoid infections and ensure stable air pressure.

- **Mask and tubing cleaning**: As with oxygen therapy, masks and tubing on non-invasive ventilation devices must be cleaned daily to remove secretions and prevent bacterial contamination. Filters should also be changed according to the manufacturer's recommendations.

- **Checking pressures** : CPAP and BiPAP machines deliver a specific air pressure to keep the airways open. It is essential to check regularly that the machine is delivering the **correct pressure**, and to recalibrate the device if necessary.

**Mechanical ventilation**

Patients on **mechanical ventilation** require particularly vigilant care due to the high risk of nosocomial infections, such as **ventilator-associated pneumonia** (VAP).

- **Circuit disinfection**: Ventilation circuits must be **disinfected** and, if necessary, **changed** regularly to prevent bacterial colonization. A strict disinfection protocol must be followed for reusable circuits, while single-use circuits must be disposed of after each use.

- **Checking filters**: The **antibacterial filters** used in mechanical ventilators play a key role in preventing infections. They must be replaced regularly, in accordance with the manufacturer's recommendations, to guarantee their effectiveness.

- **Calibrating and checking alarms**: Mechanical ventilators are equipped with **safety alarms** that warn of malfunctions such as loss of pressure or patient disconnection. These alarms should be tested regularly to ensure that they are operating correctly. Ventilation parameters, such as tidal volume and respiratory rate, also need to be checked and adjusted according to the patient's needs.

## 4. Preventing infections linked to respiratory devices

Maintaining respiratory equipment involves much more than cleaning and disinfection. It also includes a proactive approach to **infection prevention**, notably by reducing the risk of microbial colonization and training nursing staff and patients in good practices.

**Infection control protocols**

In hospital environments, specific **prevention protocols** are put in place to limit the risk of infections associated with the use of respiratory devices.

- **Patient positioning**: In ventilated patients, maintaining a **semi-seated position** (30 to 45 degrees) helps reduce the risk of **aspiration of** secretions, the main cause of ventilation-associated pneumonia.

- **Mouth care**: Regular **mouth care** with antiseptic solutions is also essential to prevent bacterial proliferation in the oropharynx, thus reducing the risk of lung infection.

**Staff and patient training**

To ensure proper use and maintenance of the equipment, it is crucial that **care staff** and, where applicable, **homecare patients** are well trained.

- **Ongoing training**: Hospital staff must be regularly trained in the latest disinfection techniques and equipment maintenance procedures. In addition, patients undergoing oxygen therapy or home ventilation must be given **clear instructions** and **practical demonstrations** on how to maintain their equipment.

  ◦ Precautions when handling devices

When **handling medical devices**, particularly those used for oxygen therapy and assisted ventilation, specific precautions must be observed to ensure the safety of patients and nursing staff. These devices are often in direct contact with the respiratory tract, making them particularly susceptible to microbial contamination. What's more, the technical nature of this equipment requires careful handling to avoid malfunctions. Here are the **main precautions to be observed** to prevent infection, ensure proper device operation and avoid accidents.

# 1. Rigorous hygiene and asepsis

The first step in handling respiratory devices is to observe **strict rules of hygiene** and **asepsis**, to limit the risk of cross-contamination between patients or with the hospital environment.

**Hand washing**

**Hand washing** is one of the most fundamental precautions when handling medical devices. It is essential before and after every procedure, whether adjusting ventilation parameters, changing masks or handling tubing.

- **Disinfection**: Use a hydroalcoholic solution or wash hands with soap and water for at least 30 seconds before touching a respirator, patient or device component.
- **Gloves**: Wear **sterile gloves** when directly handling the patient's airway or when managing invasive devices (such as endotracheal tubes). Change gloves between patients to avoid transmission of pathogens.

**Surface disinfection**

Surfaces in contact with medical equipment or patients must be **disinfected regularly**. This includes the equipment itself, side tables where equipment is placed, as well as handrails or control switches.

- **Suitable disinfectants**: Use disinfectants suited to the nature of the materials used in the devices. It is important to follow manufacturers' recommendations to avoid damage to equipment caused by the use of inappropriate products.

## 2. Handling oxygen therapy devices

Oxygen therapy involves administering oxygen to patients via **nasal cannula, oxygen masks** or **compressed oxygen cylinders**. These devices, though simple to use, require certain precautions when handled to ensure safe and effective treatment.

### Oxygen goggles and masks

- **Interface hygiene**: Oxygen goggles and masks must be handled with **clean hands** and **disinfected regularly** to prevent bacterial proliferation. They should be replaced according to the manufacturer's recommendations, or in the event of signs of deterioration (cracks, wear).

- **Secure fit**: Once the nasal **cannula** or mask is in position, it's essential to check that it fits properly to avoid **oxygen leaks**. A leak can lead to reduced treatment efficiency and potentially increase the risk of fire due to oxygen build-up.

### Handling oxygen tanks and concentrators

Pressurized oxygen tanks and **oxygen concentrators** must be handled with care to avoid accidents related to pressure or oxygen safety.

- **Safe positioning of tanks**: Oxygen cylinders should always be **stored in an upright position**, secured in suitable carts or racks to prevent them from tipping over. Never leave a tank unsecured.

- **Avoid sources of ignition**: Oxygen is a powerful oxidizer, so it's essential to keep oxygen tanks and devices away from any source of heat or ignition, including **open flames**, **electrical appliances**, or even overheated surfaces. Patients undergoing home oxygen therapy should be warned not to smoke, and to follow safety instructions.

### Humidifier management

The oxygen administered is often humidified to prevent irritation of the mucous membranes. However, **humidifiers can** become reservoirs of germs if not properly maintained.

- **Use of sterile water**: Fill humidifiers only with **sterile water** to prevent bacterial growth. Humidifiers should be emptied and disinfected daily.

- **Cleanliness check**: Inspect the humidifier regularly for deposits and signs of contamination. If the device shows signs of deterioration, it must be replaced.

## 3. Handling assisted ventilation devices

**Assisted ventilation** devices, whether **non-invasive** (CPAP, BiPAP) or **invasive mechanical ventilation**, require even more rigorous handling, given the risks of serious respiratory complications and nosocomial infections, such as **ventilation-associated pneumonia**.

### Non-invasive ventilation (CPAP and BiPAP)

Non-invasive ventilation machines, such as **CPAP** or **BiPAP**, are often used for patients suffering from sleep apnea or chronic respiratory disorders.

- **Correct mask fitting**: When handling the face or nasal mask, it's important to ensure that it fits properly to avoid **air leaks**, which can compromise treatment efficacy. The mask should not be too tight to avoid skin irritation.

- **Checking parameters**: It's vital to regularly check the **pressure settings** on CPAP or BiPAP devices. Accidental changes in settings can lead to under-ventilation or, conversely, excess pressure, which can result in barotrauma.

**Mechanical ventilation**

Patients on **mechanical ventilation** (intubated or tracheostomized) are particularly at risk of serious respiratory infections. Extra care must therefore be taken when handling breathing circuits.

- **Changing circuits**: Ventilation circuits must be changed regularly, as recommended by hospital protocols, to limit **bacterial colonization**. When replacing a circuit, take care not to touch the internal parts that will be in direct contact with the patient.

- **Disinfection of reusable devices**: Reusable parts of ventilators, such as masks and humidifiers, must be **disinfected** with suitable products between each use. Single-use components, such as antibacterial filters, must be changed after each patient.

- **Monitoring alarms**: Fans are fitted with alarms to signal faults (circuit disconnection, airway obstruction, pressure too low or too high). These alarms must be regularly tested and reset after each operation.

## 4. Staff and patient training

Correct handling of respiratory devices requires **appropriate training**, not only for nursing staff, but also for patients and their families when the devices are used at home.

**Training nursing staff**

- **Initial and ongoing training**: Hospital staff and caregivers must be trained in the proper handling of oxygen therapy and ventilation devices. This training must include not only technical management of the equipment, but also cleaning, maintenance and infection prevention procedures.

- **Practical simulations**: Organize regular **simulations** to enable caregivers to familiarize themselves with the various machines and practice safety procedures in the event of malfunction or breakdown.

## Patient and family education

For patients using home oxygen therapy or ventilation devices, it's crucial that they are well informed about how to handle these devices safely.

- **Practical demonstrations**: Caregivers should give **practical demonstrations** to show patients how to clean and maintain their equipment, adjust settings and react to problems.

- **Ongoing support**: Patients and their families must have **easy access** to resources or telephone support lines in case of doubt or difficulty when handling equipment at home.

- **Training caregivers in strict hygiene rules**
  - Hand washing, wearing protective equipment

**Hand washing** and the **wearing of protective equipment** are fundamental measures in infection prevention, particularly in healthcare environments. These practices are essential to protect both patients and healthcare staff from nosocomial infections, by limiting the spread of pathogens. Compliance with these protocols plays a key role in reducing the risk of contamination, particularly when handling medical devices or caring for vulnerable patients.

# 1. Hand washing: the first line of defense

**Hand washing** is considered one of the most effective ways of preventing the transmission of infections. It must be carried out systematically before and after each contact with a patient, before handling medical devices, and after contact with potentially contaminated surfaces or equipment.

**Hand washing methods**

There are two main ways of ensuring proper hand hygiene: washing hands with soap and water, and using hydroalcoholic solutions.

- **Washing with soap and water**: This method is recommended when hands are visibly dirty or after contact with organic substances. Washing should last **at least 30 seconds** and include rubbing all parts of the hand: palms, backs of hands, fingers, interdigital spaces, fingertips and nails.

- **Hydroalcoholic solution**: For hands that are not visibly dirty, the use of a hydroalcoholic solution is often sufficient and quicker. Rubbing should last **20-30 seconds** until hands are completely dry. Hydroalcoholic solutions are effective against most pathogens, but less effective in the presence of organic matter or bacterial spores such as *Clostridium difficile*.

**Key times for hand washing**

The WHO has defined five **key moments** when handwashing is essential in healthcare:

1. **Before touching a patient**: To avoid transferring germs to the patient.
2. **Before an aseptic procedure**: For example, before administering an injection or handling a medical device.

3. **After a risk of exposure to biological fluids**: As after touching blood, secretions or body fluids.
4. **After touching a patient**: To avoid transmitting germs to yourself or the environment.
5. **After touching the patient's environment**: Even if the patient has not been touched directly, the environment may be contaminated.

## 2. Wearing personal protective equipment (PPE)

**Wearing personal protective equipment** (PPE) is crucial to protect healthcare workers from infection when handling patients or medical equipment. PPE is particularly important for preventing cross-contamination, respiratory infections and infections caused by contact with body fluids.

### Types of protective equipment

The main protective equipment includes **gloves, masks, gowns** and **safety glasses**. Each is used in specific situations, depending on the level of risk of exposure to pathogens.

- **Gloves**: They must be worn for any handling likely to involve direct contact with body fluids, mucous membranes, open wounds or invasive medical devices (catheters, probes). Gloves must be changed between each patient and removed immediately after a procedure to avoid cross-transmission. After removing gloves, hand washing is mandatory.

- **Surgical masks**: protect against respiratory droplets emitted by patients when coughing or sneezing. They must be worn when caring for patients with respiratory infections, or when performing procedures likely to generate aerosols (such as intubation or tracheal suctioning).

- **FFP2/FFP3 masks**: These filtering masks offer a higher level of protection and are used for procedures with a high risk of airborne transmission, such as **tuberculosis**, or when caring for patients with highly contagious viral diseases such as COVID-19.

- **Gowns**: Protective gowns are used to protect the caregiver's clothing from contamination by secretions or body fluids. They are particularly necessary when providing care close to the patient, performing surgical procedures, or in intensive care units.

- **Goggles and visors**: These protect the eyes against splashes of biological fluids or aerosols. They are used during high-risk procedures or in the presence of patients with infections likely to be transmitted by droplets.

## Good practice in PPE use

Proper use of personal protective equipment is essential to its effectiveness. This includes the right fit, and how to put it on and take it off without risking contamination.

- **Correct use of masks**: A surgical mask must completely cover the mouth and nose. It is important to secure it correctly behind the ears or head, and to ensure that there are no air leaks from the sides. The mask must not be touched during use, and must be removed by the fasteners, without touching the potentially contaminated front part.

- **Change PPE between patients**: It is crucial to change gloves, masks or gowns between patients to avoid cross-transmission of infections. PPE should be disposed of in suitable containers immediately after use.

- **PPE removal**: When removing PPE, a specific sequence must be followed to avoid contact with potentially contaminated parts. For example, gloves should be removed first, followed by gowns, masks and goggles. Hands should be washed immediately after PPE removal.

# 3. Adapting precautions to clinical situations

Basic hand hygiene and PPE precautions may vary according to the **clinical context and** risk levels associated with the care to be provided.

**Standard precautions**

**Standard precautions** apply to all patients, regardless of their infectious status. They include **systematic hand washing**, wearing **gloves** whenever in contact with biological fluids or potentially contaminated surfaces, and other PPE depending on the procedure performed.

**Additional precautions**

In some cases, **additional precautions** are necessary, especially for patients with infections transmitted by air, droplets or direct contact.

- **Airborne precautions**: These precautions are applied for airborne diseases such as tuberculosis. They require the use of **FFP2/FFP3 masks** and, in some cases, the use of negative pressure chambers to prevent the spread of infectious agents in the ambient air.

- **Droplet precautions**: For illnesses such as influenza or whooping cough, **surgical masks** are used to prevent droplet transmission. Goggles or visors can be added if there is a risk of splashing.

- **Contact precautions**: These are implemented for infections transmitted by direct or indirect contact with contaminated surfaces, such as **methicillin-resistant Staphylococcus aureus (MRSA)** infections. These precautions include the wearing of **gowns** and **gloves**, and rigorous disinfection of surfaces and objects touched by the patient.

◦ Infection surveillance and control in hospitals

The **surveillance and control of hospital-acquired infections** are essential pillars in guaranteeing the safety of patients, nursing staff and all those present in a healthcare establishment. Nosocomial infections, i.e. those contracted in hospital, represent a major challenge due to their impact on morbidity, mortality, length of hospital stay and healthcare costs. These infections can affect a variety of systems, including the respiratory, urinary and blood tracts, with pathogens that are often resistant to antibiotics. Continuous surveillance, combined with rigorous infection control strategies, can reduce their incidence and improve the quality of care.

# 1. The importance of monitoring nosocomial infections

**Surveillance of** nosocomial infections is the first step in the management of these infections. It consists in collecting, analyzing and interpreting data on infections occurring in a hospital establishment, in order to detect trends at an early stage, identify risk factors, and implement appropriate corrective measures.

**Surveillance objectives**

Infection surveillance has many objectives:

- **Identifying outbreaks**: Surveillance enables us to identify nosocomial infections at an early stage, whether isolated or linked to an epidemic, so that we can take appropriate action. For example, a sudden rise in cases of ventilator-associated pneumonia in an intensive care unit may reveal a problem in respiratory device management.

284

- **Monitoring recurrent infections** : Certain nosocomial infections, such as catheter-related urinary tract infections or surgical site infections, are more frequent. Monitoring helps to detect variations in their incidence, enabling care and prevention protocols to be adapted.

- **Assessment of preventive measures**: Analysis of monitoring data enables us to assess the effectiveness of preventive measures implemented. For example, a reduction in infections after the implementation of a new disinfection procedure attests to its effectiveness.

## Monitoring methods

Monitoring methods vary according to the needs and resources of the facility, but generally include:

- **Active surveillance**: This is the regular, systematic monitoring of infections within the hospital, involving surveys of departments, analysis of medical records, and collection of data on potentially hospital-acquired infections.

- **Passive surveillance**: This type of surveillance relies on spontaneous reporting of infections by caregivers. Although simpler to implement, it can lead to under-reporting of cases if caregivers are not well trained or are overworked.

- **Infection indicators**: Standardized indicators are used to assess the incidence of nosocomial infections. For example, we calculate the rate of infections per 1,000 days of hospitalization or per 1,000 days of use of medical devices (such as catheters or ventilators).

## 2. Main nosocomial infections to watch out for

Hospital-acquired infections can affect many different organs and body systems. The most common include **surgical site infections**, **urinary tract infections**, ventilator-associated **pneumonia** and **bloodstream infections** (bacteremia) associated with medical devices. Each of these infections has its own particular characteristics and requires specific management.

**Surgical site infections (SSI)**

**Surgical site infections** occur in the surgical wound following an operation. They can be superficial, affecting only the skin, or deep, involving underlying structures such as muscles or organs.

- **Prevention**: Good management of surgical site infections relies on **strict asepsis** in the operating room, appropriate use of prophylactic antibiotics, and post-operative monitoring for signs of infection (redness, warmth, purulent discharge).

- **Monitoring**: Tracking infection rates after procedures helps to detect outbreaks of contamination or shortcomings in operating protocols.

**Catheter-related urinary tract infections**

**Urinary tract infections** are often associated with prolonged placement of **bladder catheters**, particularly in immobilized patients or those in intensive care. If left untreated, these infections can progress to **pyelonephritis** (kidney infection) or **septicemia**.

- **Prevention**: Rigorous hygiene during catheter insertion and handling, and removal of catheters as soon as possible, are key measures for preventing these infections.

- **Surveillance**: Hospital departments should monitor the rate of urinary tract infections in catheterized patients and identify high-risk practices, such as excessive device handling or the use of non-sterile catheters.

**Ventilator-associated pneumonia (VAP)**

**Ventilator-associated pneumonia** occurs in patients on prolonged mechanical ventilation. They are caused by pathogen colonization of the lower respiratory tract.

- **Prevention**: **Semi-sitting** patients, regular drainage of bronchial secretions, and maintaining good respiratory device hygiene are effective strategies for reducing the incidence of VAP.

- **Surveillance**: VAP surveillance is based on regular analysis of infections in ventilated patients, and on strict protocols for cleaning and changing ventilation circuits.

**Catheter-related bacteremia**

**Bacteremia** are bloodstream infections often associated with the use of **central venous catheters**. These infections can rapidly develop into **septicemia**, with the risk of multiple organ failure.

- **Prevention**: Sterile catheter placement, rigorous disinfection of the insertion site and regular dressing changes are essential to prevent bacteremia.

- **Monitoring**: Tracking infection rates associated with the use of venous catheters enables us to detect shortcomings in care practices or device maintenance.

# 3. Infection control strategies

**Infection control** is based on strict **health protocols** designed to prevent the spread of infectious agents. This is a multi-faceted approach, which includes hygiene measures, the appropriate use of personal protective equipment (PPE), and rigorous practices when handling medical devices.

## Hand hygiene

**Hand washing** is the simplest and most effective way of preventing nosocomial infections. It must be carried out systematically before and after every patient contact, after handling medical devices, and before aseptic procedures.

- **Washing with soap**: When in contact with biological substances, washing with soap and water is recommended.

- **Hydroalcoholic solutions**: These are used for rapid hand washing in situations where hands are not visibly soiled. These solutions reduce transient flora on hands and are effective against most pathogens.

## Use of personal protective equipment (PPE)

**Personal protective equipment** is essential to protect nursing staff and patients from infection. It includes **gloves, masks, gowns** and **goggles**.

- **Masks and gloves**: They must be worn according to the risk of contamination. **Sterile gloves** are used for invasive procedures, while **surgical masks** are worn to avoid transmission of respiratory pathogens.

- **Gowns and goggles**: Gowns are worn to protect against splashes of biological fluids, while goggles protect the eyes against splashes.

## Sterilization and disinfection of medical devices

**Medical devices** used for invasive care or in direct contact with patients must be sterilized or disinfected between uses.

- **Sterilization**: Surgical instruments and reusable devices must be **sterilized** in autoclaves or using specific methods, such as heat or chemical agents. Sterilization ensures the complete elimination of micro-organisms, including bacterial spores.

- **Disinfection**: For non-invasive surfaces and equipment, regular disinfection using suitable products (such as alcohol-, chlorine- or quaternary ammonium-based disinfectants) is essential to limit contamination.

## 4. Staff training and awareness

**Ongoing training** of hospital staff is crucial to ensure that infection prevention protocols are fully understood and applied. All caregivers, from doctors to nurses to orderlies, need to be trained in the latest infection control techniques and hygiene measures.

- **Regular training programs**: Organizing training sessions on hand washing, PPE use and medical device management helps maintain a high level of vigilance.

- **Practical simulations**: **Simulation exercises** enable caregivers to practice aseptic procedures in conditions close to reality, and to identify areas for improvement in their daily practices.

## 5. Managing epidemics in hospitals

In the event of an **epidemic** or outbreak of infection in a hospital, it is essential to react quickly to limit the spread of the infectious agent. Infection control teams must be ready to implement measures such as **patient isolation, decontamination of infected areas**, and **enhanced surveillance**.

**Isolation of infected patients**

**Isolation** is a preventive measure aimed at separating infected patients from others to prevent the spread of infections, particularly in the case of contagious diseases (influenza, tuberculosis, MRSA).

- **Isolation in a single room**: A patient with a contagious infection should be placed in a **single room**, equipped if necessary with **negative** pressure systems to prevent the spread of airborne pathogens.

- **Contact and airborne precautions**: Depending on the type of infection, **contact precautions** (wearing gloves and gowns) or **airborne precautions** (wearing FFP2 masks) must be observed by personnel.

# Chapter 11

# Respiratory rehabilitation and the role of the caregiver

- **What is respiratory rehabilitation?**
  - ◦ Rehabilitation program to improve patients' quality of life

A well-designed **rehabilitation program** aims to improve the quality of life of patients, particularly those suffering from chronic illnesses, physical limitations or who have undergone surgery. In an inpatient or outpatient setting, the program is designed to restore **physical function**, promote **autonomy**, and optimize the patient's mental and emotional health. The main aim is to enable the patient to return to **as active and independent a life as possible**, while managing symptoms and preventing complications. A rehabilitation program often encompasses a combination of **physical rehabilitation, breathing exercises, functional rehabilitation** and **psychological support**.

# 1. Rehabilitation objectives

The rehabilitation program is designed to meet the patient's specific needs, depending on his or her pathology and general condition. Main objectives include:

- **Improved physical function**: Reduce muscle loss, improve strength, flexibility and endurance, which are essential for regaining functional autonomy.

- **Optimizing respiratory capacity**: in patients with chronic lung diseases, such as **COPD** or following thoracic surgery, respiratory rehabilitation aims to improve breathing efficiency and strengthen respiratory muscles.

- **Pain management**: Many patients suffer chronic pain following trauma or surgery. Rehabilitation helps to manage this pain through specific techniques (gentle exercises, manual therapies, electrostimulation).

- **Improving autonomy**: The aim is to help patients regain their ability to perform **everyday tasks** (such as walking, dressing or climbing stairs) independently, by improving their mobility and balance.

- **Reduced anxiety and depression**: Psychological support integrated into the rehabilitation program is often necessary to help patients deal with the emotional aspects of their condition, such as frustration or fear of not regaining their former abilities.

# 2. Initial assessment and program planning

Before starting a rehabilitation program, a **comprehensive** patient **assessment** is carried out. This includes a thorough medical assessment, physical tests, a respiratory capacity analysis and a psychosocial evaluation.

### Physical and functional assessment

The physiotherapist assesses the patient's level of **mobility, muscular strength, balance** and **coordination**. This assessment is used to determine the starting point for the program, and to define short- and long-term objectives.

- **Mobility and flexibility tests**: These tests assess joint range of motion, muscle flexibility, and the ability to perform functional movements without pain.

- **Endurance assessment**: Walking tests (such as the six-minute walk test) or progressive effort tests are used to measure cardiovascular and respiratory endurance. This enables the exercise program to be tailored to the patient's exercise tolerance.

### Respiratory assessment

For patients suffering from **respiratory pathologies** such as COPD or asthma, or after thoracic surgery, a specific evaluation of respiratory functions is carried out.

- **Spirometry**: This test measures respiratory capacity and assesses the severity of bronchial obstruction, helping to adapt the rehabilitation program.

- **Pulse oximetry**: Pulse oximetry is used to monitor oxygen saturation during exercise and adapt exercise intensity to the patient's respiratory tolerance.

**Psychological evaluation**

The patient's emotional and mental state plays a crucial role in the success of a rehabilitation program. Psychological support can be offered in parallel to deal with **stress**, **anxiety** or **depression** linked to the disease or loss of autonomy.

# 3. Components of the rehabilitation program

The rehabilitation program is made up of several components, which vary according to the patient's individual needs and specific goals.

**Physical rehabilitation**

Physical exercise is at the heart of the rehabilitation program. They aim to strengthen muscles, improve cardiovascular endurance and restore mobility.

- **Muscle-strengthening exercises**: These target the main muscle groups, especially those supporting posture and functional movements (such as the quadriceps, back and abdominal muscles). They help reduce muscle weakness associated with immobility or illness.

- **Endurance exercise**: Cardiovascular training is essential to improve **general endurance** and respiratory capacity. It can include walking, cycling or treadmill exercise, depending on the patient's abilities.

- **Flexibility and balance exercises**: Stretching exercises help improve range of motion and prevent injury. Balance exercises, such as proprioception exercises, are essential to reduce the risk of falls, especially in the elderly.

**Respiratory rehabilitation**

For patients with chronic respiratory diseases or who have undergone lung surgery, respiratory rehabilitation aims to improve lung function and optimize oxygenation.

- **Controlled breathing techniques**: Techniques such as **diaphragmatic breathing** and **pursed-lip breathing** are taught to help reduce breathlessness and increase breathing efficiency.

- **Bronchial drainage**: **Controlled coughing** exercises and **postural drainage** help to evacuate secretions, which is particularly important in patients with COPD or cystic fibrosis.

- **Exercises to strengthen respiratory muscles**: Specific exercises, such as the use of **incentive spirometers**, are used to strengthen intercostal muscles and the diaphragm.

**Functional rehabilitation**

This component aims to improve patients' ability to carry out their **daily activities** independently.

- **Re-learning everyday movements**: The program includes practical activities, such as going up and down stairs, getting up from a chair, or walking on uneven surfaces, so that the patient can regain functional independence.

- **Use of technical aids**: If necessary, mobility aids (such as canes, walkers or wheelchairs) are integrated into the program, with advice on their optimal use.

**Pain management and psychological support**

Rehabilitation also includes the management of **chronic pain** through non-pharmacological methods and psychological support to help the patient overcome emotional challenges.

- **Manual therapies**: Therapeutic massage and joint mobilization techniques can help relieve pain and improve mobility.

- **Emotional support**: Rehabilitation can include psychological support to help patients manage the **stress** and **anxiety** associated with recovery, and rebuild confidence in their physical abilities.

## 4. Program monitoring and adjustments

Regular patient follow-up is crucial to assess progress, adjust exercises and ensure that objectives are met. **Periodic reassessments** enable us to monitor the patient's progress and modify the program according to his or her needs.

- **Gradual adaptation**: The program is adjusted according to the patient's progress. For example, as exercise tolerance increases, exercises can be intensified to further stimulate improvement.

- **Ongoing evaluation of objectives**: It's important to regularly review initial objectives and adjust them to reflect changes in the patient's state of health and expectations. This maintains patient motivation and ensures a personalized program.

## 5. Expected results and improved quality of life

A **well-structured rehabilitation program** offers numerous benefits to the patient's quality of life, both physically and mentally. Results vary from patient to patient, but the main improvements expected include:

- **Improved autonomy**: Patients regain the ability to carry out their daily activities without assistance or with minimal support, improving their independence and self-confidence.

- **Reduced breathlessness and improved breathing**: in patients with respiratory diseases, respiratory rehabilitation helps to better manage breathlessness and improve lung capacity, facilitating physical activity and reducing exacerbations.

- **Pain reduction**: Better pain management through physical and manual techniques improves patient comfort and reduces the need for analgesic drugs.

- **Improved mental health**: Reduced anxiety, better management of emotions and the resumption of physical activity all help to improve **mood** and reduce the **depressive** symptoms often associated with chronic illness.

  ◦ Objectives and benefits of pulmonary rehabilitation

**Pulmonary rehabilitation** is a comprehensive intervention for patients suffering from **chronic respiratory diseases**, such as **chronic obstructive pulmonary disease (COPD)**, **asthma, pulmonary fibrosis** or after **thoracic surgery**. Its main aim is to improve patients' **quality of life** by optimizing their respiratory capacity, exercise endurance and general well-being. Pulmonary rehabilitation combines **physical exercise, therapeutic education, respiratory re-education** and **psychological support** to enhance patients' autonomy and enable them to better manage the symptoms of their disease.

## Objectives of pulmonary rehabilitation

The aims of pulmonary rehabilitation are manifold, and are designed to meet the specific needs of patients. The main objectives include:

### 1. Improve respiratory capacity

Patients with chronic respiratory diseases often have **impaired lung function** and limited respiratory capacity. Pulmonary rehabilitation aims to strengthen respiratory muscles, optimize pulmonary ventilation and improve gas exchange.

- **Strengthening respiratory muscles**: Targeted exercises, such as **diaphragmatic breathing** and **breathing resistance exercises**, are designed to strengthen the diaphragm and intercostal muscles, improving the ability to inhale deeply and exhale efficiently.

- **Improved exercise tolerance**: Pulmonary rehabilitation helps to increase **exercise tolerance**, enabling patients to endure longer physical activities without suffering from severe breathlessness.

### 2. Reduce breathlessness (dyspnea)

**Shortness of breath** or **dyspnoea** is one of the most disabling symptoms for patients suffering from lung disease. Pulmonary rehabilitation aims to reduce the perception of breathlessness on a daily basis by teaching patients adapted breathing techniques.

- **Controlled breathing techniques**: Patients learn techniques such as **pursed-lip breathing**, which increases the duration of exhalation and prevents air trapping in the lungs, thus reducing breathlessness.

- **Optimizing ventilation**: Breathing exercises encourage better coordination of the respiratory muscles, maximizing the volume of air inhaled and exhaled.

### 3. Improve general fitness

Respiratory diseases often limit patients' ability to be active, leading to **physical deconditioning** (loss of muscle strength, reduced endurance). Pulmonary rehabilitation aims to reverse this physical deterioration through adapted exercise programs.

- **Muscle strengthening**: Exercises to strengthen the main muscle groups help improve the strength and function of muscles used on a daily basis (e.g. leg and trunk muscles).

- **Improving endurance**: Cardiovascular training, such as treadmill walking, stationary cycling or stair climbing, is integrated into the program to increase physical endurance.

### 4. Prevent exacerbations and hospitalization

Exacerbations (sudden worsening of respiratory symptoms) are frequent in patients with COPD or other chronic lung diseases, often leading to hospitalization. Pulmonary rehabilitation aims to reduce the frequency and severity of these exacerbations.

- **Therapeutic education**: Patients are trained to **recognize the first signs of** exacerbation and to take preventive measures, such as adjusting their treatment or calling their doctor.

- **Improved symptom management**: By learning strategies to better manage day-to-day symptoms (breathing, secretion management), patients are better prepared to prevent respiratory complications.

## 5. Promoting independence and improving quality of life

A key objective of pulmonary rehabilitation is to help patients regain their independence in daily activities, helping them overcome the physical limitations and dependency caused by their disease.

- **Improved mobility**: Rehabilitation exercises help improve patients' ability to walk, climb stairs and perform simple tasks, enabling them to regain **functional independence**.

- **Emotional and psychological support**: Living with a chronic respiratory disease can affect emotional well-being, leading to anxiety, depression or feelings of frustration. Psychological support integrated into the program helps **reduce stress** and **improve** patients' **quality of life**.

## Benefits of pulmonary rehabilitation

The benefits of pulmonary rehabilitation are well documented and affect many aspects of patients' lives. Here are some of the main benefits:

## 1. Reduced breathlessness and fatigue

Pulmonary rehabilitation helps patients to better control their breathing, thereby reducing **dyspnoea**. In addition, by strengthening respiratory muscles and improving cardiovascular endurance, it helps reduce disease-related **physical fatigue**.

## 2. Improved lung function

Although pulmonary rehabilitation cannot reverse lung deterioration caused by diseases such as COPD or pulmonary fibrosis, it can optimize the use of remaining lung capacity. Breathing exercises, in particular, improve gas exchange efficiency, helping to better **oxygenate the body**.

## 3. Increased exercise tolerance

Patients taking part in a pulmonary rehabilitation program show **improved exercise tolerance**, making it easier for them to carry out daily activities (such as walking, climbing stairs or getting dressed). This contributes to greater independence and improved quality of life.

## 4. Reduced hospitalization and exacerbations

Pulmonary rehabilitation helps prevent acute exacerbations of respiratory disease, reducing **hospital admissions** and emergency room visits. Patients are better informed and able to manage their symptoms before they worsen.

## 5. Improving mental health

Chronic respiratory diseases often affect patients' **emotional state**, causing anxiety, depression and social isolation. Pulmonary rehabilitation includes psychological support to help patients overcome these challenges, regain their self-confidence and better manage the **stress** associated with their condition.

## 6. Greater autonomy and better management of daily activities

Thanks to improved physical condition and reduced breathlessness, patients can perform the tasks of daily life more easily, improving their **independence** and their ability to maintain an active lifestyle.

- **The caregiver's role in the rehabilitation program**
  - Encourage participation in breathing exercises

Encouraging **participation in breathing exercises** is essential for patients suffering from chronic lung diseases such as **chronic obstructive pulmonary disease (COPD), asthma** and **pulmonary fibrosis**. These exercises are a key component of respiratory rehabilitation, helping to improve lung function, reduce breathlessness, and promote better day-to-day symptom management. Yet many patients are reluctant to engage fully in these exercises, often due to fatigue, lack of motivation or the perception that they are difficult or ineffective. Actively encouraging their participation therefore requires a holistic approach, taking into account physical, psychological and educational aspects.

# 1. The importance of breathing exercises

Breathing exercises are designed to strengthen the muscles involved in breathing, improve **respiratory efficiency** and reduce the sensation of **breathlessness** (dyspnoea). When practised regularly, these exercises offer numerous benefits for patients.

**Improved respiratory function**

In patients with chronic lung disease, the respiratory muscles can become weak or inefficient. Breathing exercises aim to strengthen these muscles, particularly the **diaphragm** and **intercostal muscles**, to facilitate inspiration and expiration.

- **Diaphragmatic breathing**: By encouraging deep breathing from the diaphragm, these exercises increase lung capacity and improve gas exchange.

- **Reducing air trapping**: In diseases such as COPD, air can become trapped in the lungs, making exhalation difficult. **Pursed-lip** breathing exercises help expel this stagnant air and prevent lung swelling.

### Managing breathlessness

Shortness of breath is one of the most disabling symptoms of respiratory disease. Breathing exercises teach patients to **control their breathing** in situations of stress or exertion, thus reducing the sensation of dyspnea.

- **Reducing breathing frequency**: Slow, controlled breathing techniques help to reduce breathing frequency, thus limiting breathlessness during physical activity or in stressful situations.

### Preventing exacerbations

Breathing exercises also help prevent exacerbations of respiratory illnesses, which are characterized by a sudden worsening of symptoms. By improving the efficiency of gas exchange and helping to clear secretions, these exercises reduce the risk of complications.

## 2. Factors limiting participation in breathing exercises

Despite the obvious benefits, many patients may be reluctant to take part in regular breathing exercises. This reluctance is often linked to a number of physical and psychological factors.

### Fatigue and shortness of breath

Many patients suffering from chronic lung disease experience **constant fatigue** and **severe breathlessness** at the slightest exertion. These symptoms can lead patients to avoid exercise, for fear of worsening their condition or provoking a dyspnea attack.

- **Stress-related anxiety**: Some patients develop a **fear of exertion**, fearing that breathing exercises will increase their breathlessness. This anxiety, often referred to as

**kinesiophobia** (fear of movement), can prevent them from fully engaging in their rehabilitation.

### Lack of motivation

Another common obstacle is **lack of motivation**, often linked to a lack of awareness of the benefits of breathing exercises, or a lack of immediate results. Some patients may perceive these exercises as unhelpful or too difficult to practice regularly.

### Feelings of loneliness and isolation

Chronic respiratory illness can lead to **social isolation**, limiting interaction with others and reinforcing a sense of loneliness. This can also affect patients' motivation to commit to an exercise program, especially if they lack adequate support.

## 3. Strategies to encourage participation in breathing exercises

To overcome these obstacles and actively encourage patients to participate in breathing exercises, it's important to adopt an approach that combines **education**, **motivation** and **personalized support**.

### Therapeutic education and awareness

The first step is to **inform** patients of the practical benefits of breathing exercises, explaining how they can improve their quality of life, reduce breathlessness and increase their independence.

- **Explain how exercises work**: Patients need to understand how breathing exercises work, and how they help to strengthen the respiratory muscles and oxygenate the body. It's essential to show them that these exercises can actually reduce their breathlessness in the long term.

- **Set realistic goals**: Rather than asking patients to achieve ambitious results quickly, it's important to **set modest, progressive goals**. For example, start with sessions lasting a few minutes, then gradually increase the duration and intensity of exercises.

## Psychological and emotional support

Psychological support plays a central role in motivating patients to participate in breathing exercises, especially when they feel discouraged or anxious about their disease.

- **Building self-confidence**: Patients should be encouraged to believe in their ability to perform the exercises, even if they feel tired or have difficulty breathing at first. **Regular** positive **feedback** can boost their self-confidence.

- **Managing anxiety**: by working with a psychologist or therapist, patients can learn relaxation and stress management techniques to **calmly approach** breathing exercises and avoid panic attacks in the event of dyspnea.

## Personalized coaching and support

Personalized coaching is essential to adapt breathing exercises to each patient's individual needs, taking into account their state of health and tolerance to exertion.

- **Supervision by healthcare professionals**: **Physiotherapists** or **physiotherapists specialized in** respiratory rehabilitation play a crucial role in supervising exercises. They can adapt exercise programs to the patient's abilities and provide regular follow-up to adjust sessions.

- **Home program**: For patients who are unable to visit a rehabilitation center on a regular basis, a **home respiratory exercise program** can be set up. This can include video tutorials, worksheets, or even online sessions with a professional.

- **Support groups and group rehabilitation**: Integrating patients into **rehabilitation groups** can foster a spirit of **solidarity** and **collective motivation**. Patients are more inclined to participate in exercises when they see others in similar situations progressing alongside them.

**Using technology to encourage participation**

New technologies can play a key role in encouraging participation in breathing exercises, by making them more accessible and engaging.

- **Applications and connected devices**: Specific applications enable patients to track their progress, receive reminders to exercise, and monitor parameters such as respiratory rate or oxygenation. This can increase exercise adherence by making follow-up more interactive.

- **Telerehabilitation**: **Telerehabilitation** enables patients to access respiratory rehabilitation sessions remotely, via online platforms, while benefiting from the advice of a professional. This flexible approach is particularly useful for patients living in rural areas or with mobility difficulties.

## 4. Motivate with progressive results

Once patients start to feel the benefits of breathing exercises, it's important to highlight their progress to keep them motivated. This can be done by **monitoring their performance** and showing them that they are gaining in endurance and respiratory control.

- **Measuring progress**: Keeping a **logbook** where patients record their progress (e.g. number of breaths taken, level of breathlessness before and after exercise) can help maintain motivation and visualize improvements over time.

- **Valuing small successes**: Even modest improvements, such as a reduction in dyspnea or improved ability to climb stairs, should be highlighted to encourage patients to continue their commitment to exercise.

  ○ Collaboration with physiotherapists and other professionals

**Collaboration with physiotherapists and other healthcare professionals** is essential to ensure comprehensive and effective patient care, particularly in the field of pulmonary rehabilitation and general care. This multidisciplinary approach helps to optimize care, better coordinate interventions and ensure overall monitoring of the patient's health, while meeting his or her specific needs. The **synergy between the various players in the** medical field, whether doctors, nurses, physiotherapists, psychologists or dieticians, plays a central role in improving the quality of care, preventing complications and promoting a better quality of life for patients.

# 1. The central role of physiotherapists

**Physiotherapists** play a key role in the physical and respiratory rehabilitation of patients, particularly those suffering from chronic respiratory diseases, musculoskeletal disorders or who have undergone surgery. Their expertise is fundamental to the recovery of patients' motor and respiratory functions.

**Expertise in respiratory rehabilitation**

As part of **pulmonary rehabilitation**, physiotherapists are responsible for teaching patients specific **breathing techniques**, such as **diaphragmatic breathing, pursed-lip breathing** or **controlled cough exercises**. These techniques aim to strengthen respiratory muscles, improve pulmonary ventilation and facilitate the evacuation of bronchial secretions.

- **Tailored exercise**: Depending on the patient's abilities, the physiotherapist draws up a customized exercise program, taking into account exercise tolerance, the severity of the respiratory illness and any co-morbidities. This program is regularly adjusted as the patient's condition evolves.

- **Functional rehabilitation**: For patients who have undergone thoracic surgery or are in the post-acute phase of lung disease, functional rehabilitation is an essential component. The physiotherapist guides the patient in the gradual resumption of daily activities, taking care to limit breathlessness and restore optimal physical capacity.

**Support and encouragement**

Physiotherapists also play a role in providing **psychological support**. Working closely with patients, they encourage them to persevere with their rehabilitation, even when they feel tired or discouraged. This support is essential to keep patients **motivated** and committed to regular exercise programs.

## 2. Collaboration with physicians

**Collaboration between the physiotherapist and the doctor** (whether pulmonologist, general practitioner or surgeon) is crucial to ensuring coherent care tailored to the patient's needs. The doctor assesses the patient's general condition, makes the diagnosis and prescribes the medical treatment, while the physiotherapist provides functional and respiratory rehabilitation.

**Care coordination**

Physicians and physiotherapists must communicate regularly on the patient's progress in order to coordinate care as effectively as possible. This communication enables treatments to be adjusted, therapeutic objectives to be reassessed, and the rehabilitation plan to be adapted to the patient's clinical progress.

- **Monitoring co-morbidities**: Patients with chronic diseases such as COPD or asthma often have other pathologies (diabetes, hypertension, heart failure). Collaboration between the physician and physiotherapist is essential to ensure that rehabilitation takes these co-morbidities into account, and that physical and respiratory exercises are adapted.

- **Adapting treatment**: If the physiotherapist observes signs of clinical aggravation or complications, he or she immediately informs the doctor. This makes it possible to adjust medication, modify exercises or consider additional tests.

## Preventing complications

As part of preventive care, collaboration between physicians and physiotherapists is also important in **preventing complications** linked to immobility, respiratory disease or sedentary lifestyle. For example, preventing pressure sores in bedridden patients, monitoring signs of hypoxia or managing cardiovascular risks are all areas where this synergy is essential.

# 3. Working with nurses

**Nurses** play a key role in the day-to-day care of patients, particularly in intensive care units or pneumology wards. They work closely with physiotherapists to ensure that patient care is consistent and complementary.

## Monitoring vital parameters and clinical signs

Nurses are responsible for **monitoring vital parameters** (respiratory rate, oxygen saturation, heart rate) and clinical signs in patients undergoing rehabilitation. They alert physiotherapists to any significant changes, such as an increase in dyspnea or a drop in oxygen saturation, so that exercises can be adjusted accordingly.

- **Oxygen therapy management**: Nurses work with physiotherapists to manage **oxygen therapy** or **non-invasive ventilation** devices (CPAP, BiPAP). They monitor the devices, check that oxygen is being administered correctly, and help keep patients comfortable during respiratory rehabilitation sessions.

**Preparing and accompanying patients**

Nurses often prepare patients before rehabilitation sessions, ensuring that they are in the right physical and emotional condition to perform the exercises. They can also play a role in motivating patients, encouraging them to actively participate in the exercises prescribed by the physiotherapist.

# 4. Collaboration with dieticians

**Nutrition** plays an essential role in rehabilitation, particularly for patients suffering from chronic illness or undernutrition. The **dietician** works alongside the physiotherapist to ensure that patients receive adequate nutritional intake, which is crucial for muscle recovery and improved physical endurance.

**Nutritional support**

Patients suffering from respiratory illnesses such as COPD may experience involuntary weight loss and undernutrition, aggravating breathlessness and fatigue. The dietician intervenes to adjust the diet, increasing the calorie and protein intake necessary for **muscle recovery** and **tissue repair**.

- **Nutritional follow-up**: In collaboration with the physiotherapist, the dietician assesses patients' specific nutritional needs and adjusts diets to maximize the benefits of physical rehabilitation.

## 5. Collaboration with psychologists and other health professionals

**Psychologists** and other mental health professionals (such as social workers or occupational therapists) are often involved in rehabilitation programs, particularly for patients suffering from **psychological distress**, **anxiety** or **depression**.

**Managing anxiety and motivation**

Chronic illnesses, particularly when they affect breathing and limit daily activities, can cause **significant emotional stress** for patients. Psychologists work with physiotherapists to help patients manage anxiety, overcome stress-related fears and maintain a positive attitude towards rehabilitation.

- **Psychological support**: By providing psychological support during rehabilitation, psychologists help patients to better manage their emotional symptoms, regain self-confidence and improve their mental well-being. This in turn promotes better adherence to exercise programs.

- **Social reintegration**: Social workers can also intervene to help patients **reintegrate into their social and professional lives**, providing resources and advice on available aid, support systems and access to long-term rehabilitation services.

- **Supporting the return home after long-term hospitalization**
  - Educating patients about managing their devices at home

311

**Educating patients in the management of their medical devices at home** is a crucial step in ensuring effective treatment and improving quality of life for patients with chronic diseases, particularly those requiring oxygen therapy, assisted ventilation or other respiratory support devices. When patients are discharged home after hospitalization or diagnosis, they become responsible for the use, maintenance and monitoring of these devices, which can be a challenge if they are not well prepared. Appropriate education not only helps prevent the complications associated with device misuse, but also enhances patient autonomy and engagement in their own treatment.

# 1. The importance of patient education

Managing medical devices in the home, such as **oxygen concentrators**, **nasal cannula**, **CPAP** or **BiPAP ventilators**, requires specific knowledge and skills. It is essential that patients are well informed and feel able to manage these devices independently.

### Preventing complications and errors

Improper use of medical devices can lead to serious complications, such as infections, device failure and treatment failure. For example, poor hygiene of **nasal cannula or oxygen masks** can lead to respiratory infections, while incorrectly adjusted **oxygen flow can** result in hypoxia or hyperoxia.

- **Risk management**: Training patients in the correct use of their devices reduces the risk of errors, while enabling them to recognize signs of malfunction before complications arise.

**Promoting autonomy and confidence**

When patients are properly trained to manage their devices at home, they feel more **autonomous** and develop greater **confidence** in their ability to care for themselves. This contributes to better **adherence to treatment**, as patients understand the importance of their role in the day-to-day management of their disease.

- **Sense of control**: The autonomy acquired through good device management gives patients a sense of control over their health, which is essential for reinforcing their motivation to follow therapeutic recommendations.

# 2. Teaching technical aspects

Patient training on the use of home devices needs to focus on **technical** aspects to ensure that each device is used and maintained correctly. This means providing clear, practical information and step-by-step demonstrations.

**Correct use of breathing devices**

The correct use of respiratory devices, such as **oxygen concentrators**, **nasal cannula** or **oxygen masks**, is essential to ensure that the patient receives the right amount of oxygen or pressurized air. Patients need to be trained to set certain parameters themselves, and to ensure that the device is working properly.

- **Setting the oxygen flow rate**: It's vital that the patient knows how to adjust the **flow meter** according to the medical prescription. Any unauthorized modification could result in insufficient oxygenation or oxygen overdose, with potentially serious consequences.

- **Adjusting masks and goggles**: Patients need to learn how to properly adjust their **nasal cannula** or **oxygen mask** to ensure an adequate seal and avoid leaks. An ill-fitting mask can lead to a loss of treatment efficiency, while a too-tight device can cause skin irritation or lesions.

**Device care and hygiene**

Proper maintenance of home medical devices is fundamental to preventing infections and ensuring long-term functionality. Patients need to be trained to clean their equipment regularly, and to observe the rules of hygiene.

- **Cleaning devices**: It is essential that the patient knows how to clean reusable components, such as **tubing, nasal cannula** or **masks,** to avoid the build-up of secretions or bacteria. This includes washing with soapy water, rinsing and drying before reuse.

- **Changing filters and spare parts**: Devices such as ventilators or oxygen concentrators often contain filters or parts for limited use. Patients should be trained to **replace filters** or request assistance when necessary, according to the manufacturer's recommendations.

**Monitoring and fault management**

Patients also need to be prepared to monitor the proper functioning of their devices, and to react quickly in the event of **failure** or malfunction. This includes understanding **warning signals** and **malfunction indicators**, and knowing the procedures to follow to ensure continuity of care.

- **Reacting to alarms**: Modern medical devices are equipped with alarms to signal problems, such as disconnection, inadequate pressure, or power failure. The patient must be able to recognize these alarms and follow the appropriate instructions, such as reconnecting the device or contacting technical service.

- **Emergency procedures**: In the event of a serious malfunction, such as a failure of the oxygen concentrator, the patient must know how to use a **back-up oxygen cylinder** and contact maintenance or emergency medical services.

## 3. Ongoing education and regular follow-up

Educating patients to manage their devices at home should not be limited to a single session. **Regular follow-up** and **ongoing education** are essential to ensure that the skills acquired are maintained and updated in line with changes in the patient's condition or new technologies available.

### Review and training sessions

Regular **review** and **practice** sessions are important to ensure that patients remain comfortable with managing their devices. These sessions also provide an opportunity to reassess the patient's ability to use his or her equipment and make adjustments if necessary.

- **Practical simulations**: During home visits or consultations, it can be useful to review device management protocols with the patient by carrying out **practical simulations**, such as setting up a backup oxygen cylinder or adjusting the flow rate.

### Remote monitoring and telemedicine

With the rise of **telemedicine** technologies, it is increasingly possible to provide remote monitoring of patients using home medical devices. This enables healthcare professionals to monitor vital parameters in real time, and intervene rapidly in the event of a problem.

- **Remote monitoring**: Connected devices can transmit data on oxygen saturation, respiratory rate or inspired air volume directly to medical teams, enabling precise remote monitoring and early detection of abnormalities.

**Technical support and assistance**

It is essential that the patient has access to a technical and medical **support service**, available at all times, to help with any questions or unforeseen breakdowns. A dedicated phone line or home maintenance service can provide the support needed to resolve problems quickly.

# 4. Psychological support and motivation

Beyond the technical aspect, it's also important to consider the **psychological impact** of using medical devices at home. Some patients may feel discouraged, anxious or overwhelmed by the day-to-day management of their treatment. Psychological support and appropriate motivation are essential to encourage patient adherence and commitment.

**Managing anxiety and frustration**

The continuous use of medical devices can be a source of **frustration** or **anxiety** for some patients, especially if they perceive these devices as a constraint or a constant reminder of their illness. Healthcare professionals need to support patients in managing these emotions.

- **Boosting self-confidence**: By providing positive support and acknowledging the progress made by patients in managing their devices, professionals can help boost **self-confidence** and reduce anxiety linked to the use of these devices.

**Encouraging autonomy and commitment**

The aim of home device management education is to make patients **autonomous** and **committed** to their treatment. It is important to emphasize the **benefits** of this autonomy, notably improved quality of life and greater control over the disease.

○ Advice on adapting lifestyle and physical activities
**Adjustments to lifestyle and physical activity** are essential for patients suffering from chronic diseases, in convalescence or following surgery. These adjustments are essential to improve quality of life, promote healing and reduce the risk of complications. They also enable patients to maintain their independence and general well-being, while taking into account the limitations imposed by their state of health. However, lifestyle adaptation should not be seen as a restriction, but rather as a way of optimizing one's health and living in a more balanced way, adapted to one's situation.

# 1. The importance of lifestyle adaptation

Lifestyle has a direct impact on physical and mental health. For patients suffering from chronic diseases such as **COPD**, cardiovascular disease or **diabetes**, it is crucial to adjust daily activities to limit the onset of symptoms and prevent exacerbations.

**Maintaining the balance between activity and rest**

A key aspect of lifestyle adaptation is the **management of effort and rest**. A patient must be able to maintain a balance between staying active, which is important to avoid a sedentary lifestyle and its complications, and resting sufficiently to avoid exhaustion and worsening of symptoms.

- **Avoid a sedentary lifestyle**: physical inactivity can lead to loss of muscle strength, reduced respiratory capacity, and an overall weakening of the body. Even for patients suffering from respiratory diseases such as COPD, it's essential to remain active on a daily basis.

- **Planning rest periods**: Rest should be an integral part of the day's organization, especially for people suffering from chronic fatigue or shortness of breath on exertion. Alternating between periods of activity and rest helps preserve energy and prevent fatigue attacks.

**Encouraging symptom management**

Lifestyle adaptation can also involve **behavioral adjustments** to better manage symptoms such as breathlessness, pain or fatigue. By adopting certain habits and incorporating relaxation or breathing management techniques, patients can live better on a daily basis.

- **Stress management**: Stress and anxiety can aggravate the symptoms of certain chronic illnesses. Introducing relaxation activities, such as **yoga**, **meditation** or **deep breathing** exercises, can help calm the nervous system and better manage periods of crisis.

- **Structured routines**: Having clear routines helps patients get organized and better manage their limitations. For example, scheduling difficult tasks (such as shopping or housework) at times when they feel most fit helps limit fatigue.

# 2. Adapting physical activities

For patients with chronic illnesses or in convalescence, **adapted physical activity** is a key element in maintaining good physical condition, strengthening muscles, and improving respiratory and cardiovascular capacity. Exercises must be chosen according to each patient's abilities, but movement remains essential to avoid loss of mobility and prevent complications linked to inactivity.

## Benefits of regular exercise

Physical activity has many **benefits**, even for patients with severe limitations. It stimulates the cardiovascular system, strengthens muscles, improves endurance and reduces symptoms associated with certain pathologies, such as dyspnea in respiratory diseases.

- **Improved exercise tolerance**: Patients who embark on a regular exercise program, even in moderation, often notice an improvement in their exercise tolerance. This means they can perform everyday activities with less breathlessness or fatigue.

- **Muscle strengthening**: Strengthening muscles, particularly those of the trunk and lower limbs, helps patients to maintain greater stability and limit the risk of falling. This is particularly important for the frail and elderly.

## Choosing the right activities

It is important to choose **physical activities adapted to** each patient's abilities and limitations. These exercises must be progressive, and adapted to the patient's evolving state of health.

- **Endurance exercise**: Activities such as **walking**, **stationary cycling** or **swimming** are moderate endurance exercises that promote cardiovascular and respiratory health. For patients with respiratory diseases, it's essential to start with short sessions and gradually increase the intensity.

- **Muscle-strengthening exercises**: **Light strengthening** exercises, such as using small dumbbells, resistance bands or body-weight exercises (like getting up from a chair), help maintain or improve muscle strength.

- **Flexibility and balance exercises**: Activities such as **yoga, tai chi** and gentle stretching improve flexibility, strengthen balance and help prevent joint and muscle pain.

### Adapt intensity and frequency

The intensity and frequency of physical activity should be adjusted according to each patient's effort tolerance. It is important to take into account signs of fatigue or breathlessness, so as not to push the body beyond its capacity.

- **Listening to the body's signals**: Patients need to be taught to listen to their bodies, and to stop as soon as they feel signs of excessive fatigue, pain or severe dyspnea. The aim is to engage in physical activity that improves general condition, without causing distress or overexertion.

- **Progressiveness**: For patients returning to physical activity after a period of inactivity or hospitalization, it's crucial to start gradually. Starting with a few minutes of gentle activity, then gradually increasing duration and intensity, helps to strengthen muscles and cardiovascular fitness in complete safety.

## 3. Adjustments to daily activities

Beyond formal physical exercise, lifestyle adaptation also involves **adjustments to daily activities**. This makes daily life easier and less tiring, while ensuring that the patient remains active and engaged.

### Carry out household tasks appropriately

Daily tasks such as housework, shopping and meal preparation can be exhausting for people with chronic illnesses or physical limitations. It is therefore important to adapt these tasks to make them more manageable.

- **Fragmenting tasks**: It's a good idea to divide household chores into small, manageable steps. For example, instead of doing all the housework at once, the patient can concentrate on one room at a time, with breaks between each task.

- **Using technical aids**: Technical aids, such as **walkers, grab bars** or **wheelchairs**, may be needed to help accomplish daily tasks while preserving the patient's energy. In addition, certain ergonomic household tools can make repetitive or physical tasks easier.

**Adjusting the home environment**

The home environment must be adapted to reduce unnecessary effort and maximize patient safety. Simple adjustments can make a big difference in the patient's ability to manage daily life.

- **Reorganize living spaces**: It's a good idea to place everyday objects within easy reach, avoid stairs, and create comfortable rest areas close to activity zones (such as the kitchen or bathroom).

- **Setting up a space for exercise**: Having a space at home dedicated to light exercise makes it easier for patients to engage in regular physical activity, without logistical constraints.

## 4. Social and emotional support

Lifestyle adjustments involve not only physical aspects, but also **mental and emotional well-being**. For many patients, these adjustments can be perceived as limitations or losses, and it is essential to provide psychological and social support to help them navigate these changes.

**Integrate social activities**

Maintaining social interaction is important for patients' emotional well-being, especially for those who may feel isolated because of their physical limitations. Social activities can be adapted to their state of health.

- **Adapted group activities**: Adapted social activities, such as **group walks**, **gentle gym classes** or **support groups**, help patients stay connected with others, while maintaining an active, healthy lifestyle.

**Psychological support**

For patients who find it difficult to accept lifestyle changes, or who experience frustration or depression, **psychological support** can be very beneficial.

- **Behavioral therapies**: Cognitive-behavioral therapies can help patients develop strategies to cope with their limitations, accept their condition and find new ways to maintain their emotional well-being.

# Chapter 12

# Pain management in pneumology

- **The different causes of pain in pneumology patients**
  - Chest pain associated with coughing, infections or assisted ventilation

**Chest pain** associated with coughing, respiratory infections or the use of **assisted ventilation** devices is a common symptom in patients suffering from lung diseases or requiring prolonged respiratory treatment. Although often benign, these aches and pains can be very annoying, affecting the patient's quality of life. They can occur for a variety of reasons: muscle irritation due to persistent coughing, inflammation caused by a lung infection, or discomfort associated with the use of ventilation devices. Understanding the causes of chest pain, and how to alleviate it, is crucial to improving patient comfort and recovery.

# 1. Cough-related chest pain

**Coughing** is the body's natural reflex to expel secretions and irritants from the respiratory tract. However, when it is intense, repeated or prolonged, it can cause severe chest pain, mainly of muscular origin.

**Mechanisms of cough-related pain**

**Persistent coughing** places heavy demands on the muscles of the thorax, particularly the **intercostal muscles**, which contract vigorously with each coughing effort. When these muscles are used repeatedly or excessively, they can become painful, similar to muscle soreness after intense exercise.

- **Muscle pain**: Repeated coughing episodes can lead to **muscle contractures** and intercostal pain. These pains are often felt as discomfort or a pulling sensation in the ribcage, particularly during breathing movements or extra effort.

- **Parietal pain**: Intense coughing can also irritate the **chest wall**, causing localized pain that may be mistaken for cardiac or pleural pain. They are often felt as sharp, sharp pains, accentuated during coughing episodes.

**Relieve cough-related chest pain**

To alleviate this pain, it's essential to treat both the **underlying cause of the cough** and the **muscle pain** itself. This involves :

- **Cough management**: Treating the infection or condition causing the cough (such as bronchitis or tracheitis) is a priority. **Cough suppressants** or treatments specific to the underlying disease may be prescribed to calm the cough.

- **Muscle rest**: Rest is crucial to allow the thoracic muscles to recover. Applying **heat** to the painful area can help relieve muscle tension.

- **Controlled breathing exercises**: **Diaphragmatic** or slow **breathing** techniques **can** also help relieve pressure on chest muscles and reduce discomfort.

## 2. Chest pain associated with respiratory infections

**Respiratory infections**, such as pneumonia, bronchitis or pleurisy, can be a frequent cause of chest pain. These pains often occur due to inflammation of the pulmonary structures or pleura, and can be aggravated by coughing or deep breathing.

**Causes of chest pain in respiratory infections**

Infection-related chest pain is mainly caused by **inflammation** of the lung tissue or membranes surrounding the lungs (pleura). This inflammation can irritate nerve endings in these areas, causing pain.

- **Pneumonia**: Pneumonia is a lung infection that can cause widespread chest pain, often accompanied by fever, productive cough and breathing difficulties. Chest pain is often worse during deep breathing or coughing fits.

- **Pleurisy**: Inflammation of the **pleura** (pleurisy) is a frequent cause of severe chest pain. The pleura is a thin membrane that surrounds the lungs and lines the chest wall. When this membrane becomes inflamed, it becomes painful, especially during deep breathing. The pain is often localized and described as "stabbing".

- **Bronchitis**: Bronchial infections, such as **acute bronchitis**, can also cause chest pain due to irritation of the respiratory tract. These pains are generally felt as chest tightness, aggravated by coughing.

### Management of infection-related chest pain

Treatment of chest pain associated with respiratory infections is based on **infection management** and pain relief.

- **Treatment of infection**: Antibiotics are often prescribed for bacterial infections (such as bacterial pneumonia), while viral infections (such as viral bronchitis) can be treated with antiviral drugs, if necessary. Healing the infection contributes directly to reducing chest pain.

- **Analgesics and anti-inflammatories**: To relieve chest pain, **analgesics** (such as paracetamol) or **non-steroidal anti-inflammatory drugs** (NSAIDs) may be prescribed to reduce inflammation and discomfort.

- **Postural drainage and breathing exercises**: In cases of pneumonia or bronchitis, **postural drainage** techniques or

**breathing exercises** supervised by a physiotherapist can help clear the airways and improve breathing, which can reduce the pain associated with infection.

# 3. Chest pain related to assisted ventilation

Patients requiring **assisted ventilation**, whether by **CPAP**, **BiPAP** or **mechanical ventilation**, may also experience chest pain, often due to the pressure exerted on the ribcage or the side effects of long-term treatment.

### Causes of chest pain during assisted ventilation

**Assisted ventilation** is used to improve breathing in patients suffering from respiratory failure, COPD or sleep apnea. However, the use of these devices, especially when prolonged, can lead to chest pain.

- **Pressure on the ribcage**: The use of non-invasive ventilation devices (such as CPAP or BiPAP) creates continuous pressure in the airways, which can strain the thoracic and diaphragmic muscles. This constant pressure can lead to **chest** pain or **tightness**, especially in patients who are not used to it.

- **Muscle fatigue**: Patients on mechanical ventilation may also experience **muscle pain** linked to respiratory muscle fatigue, particularly if the process of weaning off the ventilator is long or difficult.

- **Barotrauma**: In some cases, poorly adjusted mechanical ventilation or excessively high pressure levels can lead to **barotrauma** (injury caused by excessive pressure in the lungs), causing chest pain and, in more serious cases, complications such as pneumothorax.

## Management of ventilation-related chest pain

The management of chest pain associated with assisted ventilation is based on **adjusting ventilation parameters** and taking measures to relieve muscular and thoracic tension.

- **Adjusting ventilation devices**: It is essential to check **ventilator settings** regularly **to** ensure that pressure is not too high. Gradual adjustments allow the patient to become accustomed to ventilation without causing excessive pain. In the event of persistent pain, a reassessment of the ventilation strategy is required.

- **Respiratory rehabilitation**: Once the patient begins to wean off assisted ventilation, **specific breathing exercises** can help strengthen the respiratory muscles and relieve chest tension.

- **Painkillers and relaxation**: Mild **painkillers**, combined with **relaxation** or **physiotherapy** techniques, can also be prescribed to relieve chest pain and relax respiratory muscles.

○ Musculoskeletal pain due to immobilization

**Musculoskeletal pain due to immobilization** is a frequent complication in patients who spend long periods in bed, or whose mobility is restricted as a result of illness, injury or surgery. Immobilization, whether total or partial, has a profound effect on muscles, joints and bones, leading to diffuse or localized pain and loss of function. This pain can significantly affect quality of life, complicating the recovery process and making it difficult to return to normal physical activity. Appropriate, early management is essential to prevent and treat such pain, while promoting patients' functional rehabilitation.

328

# 1. Causes of immobilization-related musculoskeletal pain

Immobilization-related musculoskeletal pain is the result of a number of pathophysiological processes affecting **muscles, joints, tendons** and **ligaments**. Prolonged inactivity and lack of movement lead to structural and functional changes in body tissues.

**Muscular atrophy and weakness**

One of the main consequences of immobilization is **muscular atrophy**, which occurs when muscles are not sufficiently solicited. The absence of regular muscle contraction leads to a reduction in muscle mass and strength.

- **Reduced muscle mass**: From the very first days of immobilization, muscles begin to lose volume. This loss of muscle mass is particularly marked in the lower limbs, which can lead to general weakness and reduced mobility when activity is resumed.

- **Muscle weakness**: In addition to atrophy, immobilization leads to a **reduction in muscle strength**. Muscles become unable to support the body's weight or generate the power needed for basic movements, such as rising from a chair or walking.

**Joint stiffness and contractures**

When **joints** are not regularly mobilized, they tend to become rigid. Joint structures (cartilage, synovium) depend on movement to stay healthy. Immobilization alters this balance, leading to **joint stiffness** and **muscle contractures**.

- **Joint stiffness**: Lack of movement reduces the circulation of synovial fluid, responsible for joint lubrication. This leads to **stiffness** and loss of range of motion in the joints, especially in the hips, knees and shoulders.

- **Contractures**: Contractures occur when muscles or tendons shorten due to prolonged immobilization. Patients may develop painful **muscle contractures**, which further limit their mobility.

### General deconditioning

Immobilization not only affects muscles and joints, but also the entire **musculoskeletal** and cardiovascular **system**. The resulting general **physical deconditioning** reduces endurance capacity and aggravates musculoskeletal pain on resumption of activity.

- **Osteopenia and osteoporosis**: Prolonged immobilization reduces bone density, particularly in the elderly. The lack of load on the bones can lead to **osteopenia** and even **osteoporosis**, increasing the risk of fractures.

- **Diffuse pain**: Physical deconditioning often leads to **widespread** pain throughout the body, particularly in muscles that have not been used, as well as pain linked to poor posture or prolonged bed rest.

## 2. Frequent localization of musculoskeletal pain

**Musculoskeletal pain linked to immobilization** can affect several parts of the body, with a particular prevalence in certain areas depending on the prolonged position or mechanical stress to which the body is subjected.

### Back and spine pain

The **back** is often a major area of pain in immobilized patients, due to the pressures exerted on the spine and paravertebral muscles during bed rest or prolonged poor posture.

- **Lower back pain**: Immobilization can lead to lower back pain (lumbago), due to reduced tone of the spinal stabilizing muscles and inactivity. The **intervertebral disc** is less hydrated during inactivity, which increases the risk of pain and disc herniation.

- **Cervicalgia**: Neck pain is also common, especially if the head position is not properly adjusted. Patients may develop muscle tension and stiffness in the neck region, exacerbated by inactivity.

## Lower limb pain

The **lower limbs**, especially the hips, knees and ankles, are particularly vulnerable to immobilization, due to rapid loss of muscle mass and joint stiffness.

- **Hip pain**: Prolonged immobilization often leads to **hip pain**, especially if the patient is bedridden or sitting for long periods. Loss of mobility in the hips can limit the ability to stand up or walk.

- **Knee pain**: The **knees** are also affected by muscle stiffness and contracture, particularly in the quadriceps and hamstring muscles. This stiffness can lead to pain when flexing and extending the knee, and limit walking.

## Upper limb pain

The **upper limbs**, although less often called upon in basic physical activities, can also be affected by prolonged immobilization, particularly in the shoulder and wrist areas.

- **Shoulder pain**: the shoulders, which are often little used during periods of immobilization, can become stiff and painful. **Scapulohumeral periarthritis** (inflammation of the tendons around the shoulder) can occur as a result of inactivity and prolonged positioning of the arms in the same posture.

- **Wrist pain**: In some cases, patients who are bedridden or have limited mobility may develop **wrist pain**, due to pressure exerted on the joints when they lean on their arms or use mobility aids.

# 3. Managing musculoskeletal pain

The management of musculoskeletal pain associated with immobilization is based on a **preventive** and **therapeutic** approach, aimed at maintaining mobility, preventing muscle atrophy and joint stiffness, while offering pain relief.

**Early mobilization and adapted physical exercises**

**Early mobilization** is one of the most effective ways of preventing immobilization-related musculoskeletal pain. Even if the patient cannot move independently, light exercises or passive movements performed by healthcare professionals can help maintain joint flexibility and muscle strength.

- **Passive exercises**: For patients who can't move on their own, **passive exercises** (where a caregiver or physiotherapist performs the movements) help maintain joint mobility and avoid stiffness. These movements can include joint flexion and extension, as well as gentle rotations.

- **Active exercise**: For more independent patients, it is essential to carry out **active exercises**, even light ones, to maintain muscle strength. Regular, progressive **stretching exercises** help preserve joint range of motion and avoid contractures.

## Physiotherapy and manual therapies

**Physiotherapy** plays a crucial role in the treatment of musculoskeletal pain. Techniques such as **massage, joint mobilization** and **assisted stretching** relieve pain and improve circulation, helping to prevent stiffness and muscle tension.

- **Therapeutic massage**: Gentle massages of muscles and joints help relax tight muscles, reduce inflammation and stimulate blood circulation, improving flexibility and recovery.

- **Heat or ice therapy**: Applying **heat** to painful areas releases muscle tension and improves circulation. Conversely, **cryotherapy** (application of ice) can help reduce inflammation and acute pain.

## Pain management

To relieve the musculoskeletal pain associated with immobilization, medication may be prescribed alongside physical interventions. **Analgesics** (such as paracetamol) and **non-steroidal anti-inflammatory drugs** (NSAIDs) are often used to reduce pain and inflammation.

- **Analgesics**: Paracetamol or mild opioids can be prescribed for moderate to severe pain. A cautious approach is needed to avoid dependence on opioid analgesics in patients with chronic pain.

- **Infiltrations**: In some cases, corticosteroid **infiltrations** may be considered to reduce inflammation in particularly affected joints, such as the knees or shoulders.

- **Non-drug pain management strategies**
  - Relaxation techniques, managing patient positioning

**Relaxation techniques** and the **management of patient positioning** are essential aspects in the management of patients suffering from chronic pain, disease-related stress or physical limitations due to immobilization. These approaches help to relieve pain, reduce stress and prevent complications associated with poor posture, such as pressure sores or muscle contractures. By combining relaxation and good positioning, caregivers can significantly improve patient comfort and quality of life, while promoting recovery.

# 1. Relaxation techniques to reduce pain and stress

**Relaxation techniques** aim to reduce muscular tension, calm the nervous system and reduce stress levels in patients. These techniques are particularly beneficial for people suffering from chronic illness, musculoskeletal pain or stress related to hospitalization or rehabilitation. By relaxing the mind and body, patients can better manage pain and improve their exercise tolerance.

**Progressive muscle relaxation**

**Progressive muscle relaxation** is a technique that involves progressively contracting and then releasing different muscle groups in the body. This method helps you to become aware of tensions in the body and to release them.

- **Steps** : The patient is invited to settle into a comfortable position, usually lying down. He/she begins by contracting a muscle group (e.g., the foot muscles), holds this contraction for a few seconds, then releases completely. This technique is repeated for each muscle group, from the feet to the head.

- **Benefits**: By releasing accumulated muscular tension, this method reduces musculoskeletal pain, improves blood circulation and provides an overall feeling of relaxation. It is particularly useful for patients suffering from chronic pain or immobilization-related stress.

## Diaphragmatic breathing and breath control

**Diaphragmatic** or **deep breathing** is a simple and effective technique for calming the nervous system and reducing tension. It is particularly useful for patients suffering from **dyspnea** (difficulty breathing), stress or anxiety.

- **Technique**: The patient is encouraged to take slow, deep breaths, using the diaphragm rather than the chest. Exhalation should be slow and controlled, sometimes with the lips pursed to prolong exhalation. This technique lowers respiratory rate and improves oxygenation.

- **Benefits**: By reducing respiratory effort and improving oxygenation, diaphragmatic breathing helps reduce tension in the respiratory muscles, relieves breathlessness and provides mental and physical relaxation. It is particularly beneficial for patients suffering from **COPD**, asthma or heart disease.

## Guided visualization and meditation

**Guided visualization** and **meditation** are mental relaxation techniques that help divert attention from pain or stress by focusing on soothing images or positive sensations.

- **Visualization**: Patients are invited to close their eyes and imagine a peaceful place, such as a beach or forest. The aim is to immerse oneself in this mental image, concentrating on sensory details (sounds, colors, tactile sensations). This technique helps induce a state of calm.

- **Meditation**: By concentrating on the breath or repeating a soothing word or phrase, meditation calms the mind and reduces anxiety. It also helps reduce the perception of pain and promotes general relaxation.

- **Benefits**: These techniques are particularly useful for patients suffering from chronic pain, stress or depression. They help improve **resilience** in the face of pain and enhance **mental well-being**.

**Massage therapy**

**Therapeutic massage** is a physical technique designed to relax tense muscles, improve blood circulation and reduce musculoskeletal pain. It can be performed by professionals, such as physiotherapists, or be simple and localized for comfort.

- **Techniques**: Massage can include light pressure on painful areas, circular movements to stimulate blood circulation or gentle stretching to improve muscle flexibility.

- **Benefits**: Massage helps reduce muscular tension and improve comfort in bedridden or immobilized patients. It also promotes better recovery after injury or surgery.

# 2. Managing patient positioning to prevent complications

Patient **positioning**, whether **ridden-bed** or in a wheelchair, plays a key role in preventing **complications associated with immobilization**, such as **pressure sores**, **muscle contractures** and **breathing difficulties**. Good positioning not only relieves pain, but also facilitates breathing, promotes blood circulation and prevents joint stiffness.

**Prevent pressure sores and pressure points**

**Pressure sores** occur when the skin is subjected to prolonged pressure, particularly in immobilized patients. **Regular and varied positioning** is essential to avoid these complications.

- **Frequent change of position**: We recommend **changing the** patient's **position** every 2 to 3 hours to spread the pressure over different parts of the body. This relieves pressure in high-risk areas (heels, sacrum, hips) and helps prevent pressure sores.

- **Use of cushions and supports**: Positioning cushions, **anti-bedsore mattresses** and **footrests** are important tools for improving patient comfort. For example, placing cushions under the heels to raise them slightly reduces pressure on these vulnerable areas.

**Positioning to facilitate breathing**

**Positioning** also has a direct impact on **breathing**. For patients with **breathing difficulties** (such as COPD or heart failure patients), good posture can facilitate lung expansion and improve oxygenation.

- **Semi-sitting position**: A **semi-sitting position** (or Fowler position) with the back slightly inclined at 30 or 45 degrees is ideal for facilitating breathing. This helps to relieve pressure on the diaphragm and improve oxygenation in patients suffering from respiratory insufficiency.

- **Lateral position**: In the event of breathing difficulties, it is often beneficial to **turn the patient on his or her side** to relieve pressure on the lungs and allow better drainage of pulmonary secretions. This is particularly useful for patients suffering from pneumonia or bronchitis.

**Positioning to prevent contractures and stiffness**

Prolonged poor positioning can lead to **joint contractures** and **stiffness**, particularly in bedridden patients. These complications can limit mobility and lead to chronic pain.

- **Joint alignment**: It's important to ensure that **joints** (such as hips, knees and shoulders) are properly aligned. For example, when lying down, placing a cushion under the knees can reduce tension in the lumbar muscles and prevent hip stiffness.

- **Use of soft immobilization supports**: To prevent contractures, **splints** or **ergonomic cushions** can be used to hold limbs in a functional position without causing stiffness. This is particularly important for patients who have difficulty moving themselves.

**Encouraging passive and active mobility**

Even when immobilized, it's important to encourage patients to perform **passive** or **active** movements to keep muscles and joints supple.

- **Passive movements**: Caregivers can gently mobilize the patient's limbs to perform passive movements. This helps maintain joint flexibility and prevent stiffness.

- **Active movements**: Whenever possible, encouraging the patient to perform small **active movements**(such as flexing and extending the ankles or wrists) helps stimulate circulation and maintain muscle strength.

# 3. Combining relaxation and good positioning for optimum comfort

The combination of **relaxation techniques** and **proper positioning** creates an environment conducive to recovery, comfort and pain management. These two approaches complement each other to help the patient find a position that relieves pressure and pain, while encouraging physical and mental relaxation.

- **Relaxation in optimum position**: When the patient is well positioned, relaxation techniques such as diaphragmatic breathing or guided visualization become more effective. The patient is then able to release tension in the muscles and breathe more easily, promoting a state of deep relaxation.

- **Positioning to improve sleep**: Good positioning is also crucial for improving **sleep quality** in patients. Comfortable positioning, combined with relaxation techniques before bedtime, can help reduce nocturnal pain and promote restful sleep.

　　　　○　　Psychological support and active listening
**Psychological support** and **active listening** play an essential role in the overall care of patients, especially those suffering from chronic illnesses, persistent pain or going through periods of emotional vulnerability, such as prolonged hospitalization or rehabilitation after trauma. These two complementary approaches not only bring emotional comfort to the patient, but also create a bond of trust with the care team, facilitating better adherence to treatment and a more serene recovery. Psychological support aims to help patients manage their emotions, while active listening is a communication method that encourages patients to express themselves, helping them to feel understood and respected.

# 1. The importance of psychological support in the context of care

**Psychological support** is an essential component of care, as a patient's emotional state has a direct impact on his or her general well-being and ability to cope with illness. Faced with chronic or serious pathologies such as cancer, respiratory disease or heart disease, many patients may experience anxiety, depression, fear or uncertainty about their future. Psychological support is designed to help patients manage these emotions more effectively and live with their illness more serenely.

**Help overcome anxiety and fear**

**Anxiety** is a common feeling among patients faced with a serious illness or heavy treatment. Fear of the future, fear of pain or complications, and uncertainty about the outcome of treatment can generate intense stress. Psychological support helps patients understand their emotions and learn to manage them more effectively.

- **Personalized support**: By offering a space for free expression, caregivers or psychologists can help patients express their fears and receive clear answers, which often reduces anxiety linked to the unknown.

- **Stress management techniques**: Methods such as relaxation, meditation or deep breathing are often incorporated into psychological support to help calm the nervous system and reduce anxiety.

**Support for depression and discouragement**

**Depression** and **discouragement** are also common in patients undergoing prolonged periods of treatment or coping with incurable illnesses. In these situations, psychological support can bring comfort, boost self-esteem and encourage a more positive perception of the situation.

- **Building self-esteem**: Psychological support helps restore patients' self-confidence, showing them that they are capable of overcoming the challenges of their illness. This often means encouraging them to take an active part in their treatment, and to value the little successes they achieve every day.

- **Resilience support**: trained psychologists or caregivers can teach patients techniques to develop their **resilience**, i.e. their ability to bounce back from adversity, by focusing on their strengths and coping skills.

**Managing emotional upheaval**

Serious or chronic illness often leads to **emotional upheaval**, which can affect not only the patient, but also those close to him or her. Illness often disrupts family and social equilibrium, generating tensions, misunderstandings and conflicts. Psychological support can help patients and their families cope with these challenges.

- **Supporting loved ones**: Psychological support doesn't stop with the patient; it also extends to his or her family, who may be faced with feelings of fear, helplessness or exhaustion. Offering loved ones a place to listen and share helps them better understand their needs and support them in their role as caregivers.

- **Managing emotions**: Patients may feel overwhelmed by conflicting emotions such as anger, sadness or frustration. Psychological support helps them to explore these feelings, accept them and channel them constructively.

## 2. Active listening: an essential method for understanding and support

**Active listening** is an indispensable method of communication in healthcare, as it creates a bond of trust between patient and caregiver, while fostering a deep understanding of the patient's needs, fears and expectations. It implies total attention to what the patient is saying, without judgment, and a willingness to understand his or her emotions and experience.

## The principles of active listening

Active listening is based on several principles that help establish a relationship of trust and facilitate patient expression. It requires an **empathetic** attitude, i.e. the ability to put oneself in the patient's shoes, to feel what he or she is going through, and to accept him or her as he or she is.

- **Total presence**: When practicing active listening, it's essential to concentrate fully on the patient, avoiding distractions, maintaining eye contact and adopting an open, receptive posture. This shows the patient that his or her words are important and taken seriously.

- **Rephrasing**: To make sure they've understood the patient's message, caregivers can rephrase what they're saying. This not only clarifies any misunderstandings, but also shows the patient that he or she is being listened to and understood.

- **Non-judgment**: Active listening implies a total absence of judgment. The caregiver must welcome the patient's words, without criticizing or minimizing his or her emotions, even if they seem irrational or disproportionate.

## The impact of active listening on the patient

Active listening has a **profound impact** on patients' well-being, enabling them to feel heard and supported in an environment where they can freely express their anxieties, doubts and needs. It also fosters a sense of **emotional security**, essential for creating a climate of trust in the caregiver-patient relationship.

- **Encouraging emotional expression**: Many patients find it difficult to talk about their emotions, whether for fear of disturbing others or because they feel misunderstood. Active listening creates a space where patients feel confident enough to share their fears, pain or frustrations.

- **Reducing anxiety**: The simple fact of being able to express oneself fully without being interrupted or judged can have a calming effect on patients. By verbalizing their worries, they feel less alone in the face of their illness, and more supported by the care team.

**Active listening techniques**

To practice active listening effectively, certain specific techniques can be used to encourage dialogue and deepen understanding of the patient's needs.

- **Ask open-ended questions**: Open-ended questions, which can't be answered with a simple "yes" or "no", encourage the patient to express themselves further. For example, instead of asking "Are you all right?", you can say "How are you feeling today?

- **Reflecting emotions**: The caregiver can also reflect the patient's emotions by rephrasing what he or she has said, while expressing empathy. For example: "I hear that this situation is causing you a lot of stress. Tell me a little more about what's worrying you."

- **Caring silence**: Sometimes silence is a powerful form of active listening. It allows patients to reflect and express themselves at their own pace, without pressure. The caregiver must respect these moments of silence, while remaining present and attentive.

# 3. Integrating psychological support and active listening into clinical practice

Integrating **psychological support** and **active listening** into care requires a collaborative, holistic approach, with each member of the care team contributing to the patient's overall care. This means recognizing the importance of the emotional and mental aspects of the healing process, and ensuring a safe, empathetic environment.

## Patient-centered care

The **patient-centered care** approach places the patient's needs, preferences and emotions at the heart of care. By combining psychological support and active listening, caregivers create a space where patients feel valued and understood.

- **Personalizing support**: Every patient is unique, and it's essential to tailor psychological support to his or her personal situation, beliefs and expectations. Active listening provides valuable information on patient preferences, helping to personalize care.

- **Strengthening communication within the team**: Good communication between the different members of the care team is essential to ensure consistent psychological support. Information shared during exchanges with the patient must be passed on smoothly to avoid misunderstandings and ensure appropriate care at every stage.

## Long-term support

For some patients, especially those with chronic illnesses, the need for psychological support and active listening is long-term. It's important to maintain regular follow-up and provide a space where patients can continue to express their feelings, even after treatment has ended.

- **Ongoing psychological monitoring**: Regular consultations with a psychologist or caregiver trained in active listening can help monitor the patient's emotional development and provide long-term support in managing the psychological aspects of the disease.

- **Monitoring and adjusting analgesic treatments**
  - The caregiver's role in detecting pain

The **caregiver's role in detecting pain** is fundamental to ensuring quality patient care, particularly in hospitals, long-term care facilities or at home. Often in front-line contact with patients, the caregiver is in a privileged position to observe, listen and detect signs of pain, sometimes not expressed verbally. Their vigilance, attention to detail and proximity to patients make them a key player in the early recognition of pain, enabling rapid and effective intervention to improve the comfort and well-being of those being cared for.

# 1. The importance of early pain detection

**Early detection of pain** is essential to prevent it from becoming chronic or worsening, leading to further complications. Pain, whether acute or chronic, physical or psychological, has a profound impact on a patient's quality of life. When pain is misjudged or ignored, it can impede recovery, cause emotional distress, and reduce adherence to treatment. The caregiver, by being close to the patient in his or her daily care, plays a central role in this detection.

**Unexpressed pain: a challenge**

It's important to recognize that **not all patients will verbalize their pain**. Some, out of modesty, fear of disturbing others or lack of communication, will not explicitly say that they are in pain. This is particularly true of elderly patients, children, people with cognitive impairments, or those who have difficulty expressing themselves, such as after a stroke. In these situations, the caregiver's ability to **detect non-verbal signs** of pain becomes crucial.

## 2. Observing and recognizing signs of pain

The caregiver must use observation and communication skills to identify the **physical** and **behavioral signs** that the patient is in pain. These signs may vary according to the intensity and nature of the pain, and the patient's ability to express it.

**Physical signs of pain**

Certain **physical signs** are often indicative of pain, even when the patient is not complaining directly. Caregivers, who are in regular contact with the patient for hygiene, mobility or feeding, can spot these signs.

- **Facial mimics**: The face is a valuable indicator of pain. Tense, grimacing expressions, furrowed brows or pursed lips can be clues to suffering.

- **Body position or posture**: A patient who adopts an abnormal position or stands unusually still may try to avoid moving to avoid triggering pain. For example, a patient suffering from abdominal pain may withdraw into himself/herself, while a patient with joint pain may avoid moving certain limbs.

- **Breathing changes**: **Rapid**, irregular or shallow **breathing** may be a sign that the patient is in pain, particularly in the case of chest or abdominal pain. Shortness of breath or gasping may also be linked to acute pain.

- **Muscle tension**: The body often reacts to pain with **involuntary muscle contraction**. The patient may clench his or her fists, stiffen up, or show signs of tension in the shoulders or back.

**Behavioral signs of pain**

In addition to physical signs, the caregiver needs to be alert to **behavioral changes** that may indicate the patient is in pain. A patient's behavior may change subtly or more markedly in response to pain.

- **Irritability or restlessness**: A patient who suddenly becomes irritable, restless or difficult to manage may be suffering from unexpressed pain. Agitation may also manifest itself in repeated movements, such as constantly changing position in bed or pawing at the covers.

- **Lethargy or withdrawal**: Conversely, pain can also cause some patients to withdraw into themselves. They may become **quieter**, less responsive to stimuli, or show a loss of interest in daily activities, such as eating or interacting with caregivers.

- **Decreased appetite**: Sudden loss of appetite or refusal to eat can also be a sign of pain, particularly in cases of abdominal or gastrointestinal pain.

**Indirect verbal expressions**

Even if patients don't explicitly say they're in pain, they may leave **indirect verbal clues** that betray suffering. Phrases such as "I feel tired", "I'm not comfortable" or "I have trouble moving" can mask underlying pain. The caregiver must be attentive to these phrases and interpret them in the patient's general context.

## 3. Tools and techniques for assessing pain

Caregivers can use a variety of **pain assessment tools** to better understand the intensity and nature of the pain experienced by the patient. These tools are often based on scales that enable the patient to give an estimate of his or her pain, or on observation grids for patients who are unable to express themselves.

**Pain assessment scales**

**Pain assessment scales** are simple, accessible tools for measuring the intensity of pain experienced by patients.

- **Numerical scale**: This is a scale in which the patient is asked to **rate his or her pain** on a scale from 0 to 10, where 0 represents the absence of pain and 10 the most intense pain imaginable. This method is often used with patients who are able to communicate verbally.

- **Visual Analog Scale (VAS)**: The VAS consists of a scale on which patients indicate the intensity of their pain, ranging from "no pain" to "maximum pain". This tool is particularly useful when the patient is uncomfortable with numbers.

- **Face scale**: This scale shows a series of faces ranging from a smiling face (no pain) to a crying face (intense pain). It is often used for children or people who have difficulty expressing themselves.

**Behavioral observation grids**

For non-communicative or cognitively impaired patients, **behavioral observation grids** can be used by the caregiver to assess pain based on observable signs.

- **Algoplus Grid**: This tool is designed for non-communicative elderly patients. It assesses behaviors such as facial expression, responses to care, movements or vocalizations, to determine whether the patient is in pain.

- **Doloplus 2**: Used for patients with dementia or cognitive impairment, this grid identifies pain through behavioral, somatic and psychosocial signs.

## 4. Communicate with the care team

Once pain has been detected, it is crucial that the caregiver communicates his/her observations to the **nursing team** or **physician** so that appropriate action can be taken. The caregiver must report not only the intensity of the pain, but also its location, its nature (burning, stabbing, pressure, etc.) and the factors that aggravate or alleviate it.

### Information transmission

The nursing auxiliary plays an essential role in **transmitting information** to the medical team. They must promptly report any newly detected pain, or any change in the intensity of known pain, so that treatment adjustments can be considered.

- **Clarity and precision**: The caregiver must be precise in his or her descriptions, reporting observations clearly and indicating the specific times or circumstances in which the pain occurred.

- **Continuity of care: Continuity of care** is facilitated by good communication between team members. If a caregiver changes shift or department, he or she must ensure that information on the patient's pain status is passed on to the next shift.

## 5. The role of active listening in pain assessment

In addition to observation, the caregiver must **actively listen to** encourage the patient to express his or her pain. By establishing a climate of trust, the caregiver enables the patient to feel comfortable enough to talk about his or her suffering without fear of being judged or ignored.

**Building trust**

Active listening requires an empathetic, attentive and non-judgmental attitude. The caregiver must ask open-ended questions and show genuine interest in the patient's feelings.

- **Encouraging dialogue**: by asking questions such as "How are you feeling today?" or "What's bothering you most at the moment?", the caregiver opens up a space of expression for the patient, who can feel confident to talk about his or her pain.

- **Respond with empathy**: It's important to validate the patient's emotions by showing empathy. Phrases like "I understand how difficult this must be" or "Thank you for telling me this, I'll talk to the nurse" reinforce the feeling of being heard.

  ◦ Communication with medical team for dose adjustment

**Communicating with the medical team to adjust doses** is a crucial step in patient care, particularly when it comes to drug treatments designed to relieve pain, treat infection or manage chronic disease. The effectiveness and safety of treatments depend to a large extent on close collaboration between the various members of the healthcare team, including the nurse, doctor, pharmacist and other members of the team, such as care assistants. Clear, precise and structured communication ensures that drug doses are correctly adjusted to take account of changes in the patient's state of health, therapeutic response and possible side effects.

# 1. Importance of dose adjustment

Adjusting drug doses is often necessary to optimize a patient's treatment and ensure its **efficacy**, while minimizing the **risk of**

**side effects** or toxicity. Indeed, response to drug therapy is not linear and can vary according to a number of factors, such as age, weight, renal function, drug tolerance and disease progression.

## Therapeutic response

A patient may not respond optimally to a standard dose of medication. For example, in pain management, the dose of an **analgesic** may be insufficient to effectively control pain. In such cases, dose adjustment is essential to improve patient comfort and ensure a better quality of life.

- **Evaluation of efficacy**: If the patient continues to experience severe pain despite taking medication, it is necessary to adjust the dose to obtain adequate relief. This may involve increasing the dose, changing the frequency of administration or combining different medications.

## Managing side effects

Conversely, some patients may develop **undesirable side-effects** associated with too high a dose or increased sensitivity to certain drugs. These side effects, such as nausea, vomiting, excessive drowsiness or gastrointestinal disorders, can reduce adherence to treatment and adversely affect the patient's well-being.

- **Dose reduction**: When side effects appear, it may be necessary to reduce the dose of the drug to avoid complications while maintaining sufficient therapeutic effect.

## Adjustment for comorbidities

**Co-morbidities**, such as renal, hepatic or cardiac insufficiency, can affect the way the body metabolizes and eliminates drugs. In these cases, dose adjustments are often necessary to avoid dangerous accumulation of the drug in the body, which could lead to toxicity.

## 2. Role of different members of the medical team

Dose adjustment is a collaborative process involving active communication between all members of the healthcare team. Each healthcare professional plays a specific role in this process, and coordination between them is essential to ensure rapid, safe dose adjustment.

**The nurse's role**

**Nurses** are often at the forefront of monitoring patients on medication. They are responsible for administering medication, assessing vital signs, observing drug effects and communicating this information to the medical team.

- **Monitoring and follow-up**: The nurse monitors the evolution of the patient's symptoms and notes any side effects or complications. They play a key role in **monitoring** treatment **efficacy** (e.g., pain reduction, improvement in respiratory parameters) and identifying signs of over- or under-dosing.

- **Regular reporting**: When dose adjustments are necessary, the nurse reports to the physician or pharmacist to discuss possible treatment modifications. He/she is also responsible for **checking doses** before administration, especially in situations where doses need to be adjusted regularly, such as infusion or injection treatments.

**The doctor's role**

The **doctor** is the main decision-maker when it comes to adjusting doses. He relies on the observations of the care team, the results of clinical and biological examinations, and his own expertise to adjust prescriptions.

- **Clinical assessment**: Depending on the information provided by the healthcare team (in particular, clinical signs and observed side effects), the doctor may decide to increase or decrease the dose, change the medication or combine different therapeutic options.

- **Consultation with the pharmacist**: For certain complex prescriptions, such as those involving multiple drugs or adjustments for polypharmacy patients, the physician can work closely with the pharmacist to assess drug interactions and determine the most appropriate dose.

## The pharmacist's role

The **pharmacist** plays a key role in dose adjustment, ensuring the safety of prescriptions and checking for potential drug interactions. They also provide recommendations on dose adjustment, taking into account factors such as the patient's renal or hepatic function.

- **Dose calculation**: For certain drugs, such as antibiotics, anticoagulants or potent analgesics, the pharmacist can calculate doses according to **individual** patient **parameters**, such as weight, body surface area or renal clearance.

- **Preventing interactions**: The pharmacist also reviews all prescribed medications to ensure that they are compatible, and that no dangerous interactions are likely to worsen the patient's condition.

## The caregiver's role

Although the caregiver is not directly involved in prescribing or administering medication, he or she plays a crucial role in

**detecting clinical signs** that may indicate the need for dose adjustment.

- **Patient observation**: The caregiver is often the one who spends the most time with the patient on a daily basis. He or she is therefore in a position to observe subtle changes in behavior, signs of pain, drowsiness, agitation or discomfort that could signal a treatment-related problem. These observations are essential for informing the care team and facilitating rapid dose adjustment.

- **Communication with the nurse**: By passing on this information to the nurse or doctor, the caregiver contributes to informed decisions on dose management.

## 3. Communication process to adjust doses

**Fluid, clear communication** between all members of the medical team is essential for effective dose adjustment. This process requires constant vigilance and the transmission of precise information.

**Reporting clinical signs**

One of the most important roles of the healthcare team is to promptly report **clinical changes** in the patient that may require dose adjustments. This includes such things as:

- Decreased or increased efficacy of treatment (e.g. persistent pain despite analgesics).
- The appearance of side effects, such as nausea, skin rashes, digestive disorders or signs of overdose (drowsiness, confusion).
- Abnormalities in vital signs, such as heart rate, blood pressure or oxygen saturation.

This information must be communicated immediately to the doctor and pharmacist so that decisions can be made about dose adjustment.

### Interdisciplinary communication

**Interdisciplinary communication** between team members is crucial. It needs to be structured and regular, especially during shift changes or clinical meetings.

- **Transmission of information**: When transmitting information between caregivers (e.g. between day and night shifts), it is essential that information on ongoing dose adjustments, clinical observations and patient reactions is accurately conveyed.

- **Team meetings**: Regular meetings between the entire care team (doctors, nurses, pharmacists, orderlies) enable us to review the patient's condition, assess response to treatment and adjust doses if necessary.

### Documentation of adjustments

Each dose change must be accurately **documented** in the patient's medical record. This includes the reasons for the adjustment, the new doses prescribed and the therapeutic objectives pursued. Good documentation ensures that all team members have access to the information they need to ensure continuity of care.

## 4. Monitoring and reassessment

Dose adjustment is not a static process. It requires **ongoing monitoring** to ensure that changes in treatment are producing the desired effects without causing complications.

### Continuous monitoring

After each dose adjustment, close monitoring of the patient's **response to treatment** is necessary. This includes assessment of symptoms, monitoring of side effects and, if necessary, biological tests (e.g., blood drug assays for treatments with narrow therapeutic margins).

**Regular re-evaluation**

**Regular reassessment of** treatment is essential to adjust doses in line with changes in the patient's clinical condition. This ensures that the therapeutic strategy remains adapted to the patient's needs and state of health.

# Chapter 13

# The role of the caregiver in the care of patients with rare respiratory pathologies

- **Overview of rare lung diseases**
  - Idiopathic pulmonary fibrosis, sarcoidosis, pulmonary hypertension

**Idiopathic pulmonary fibrosis**, **sarcoidosis** and **pulmonary hypertension** are three chronic respiratory diseases with different mechanisms, but which share serious consequences for lung function and patient well-being. These pathologies, often complex to diagnose and treat, have a major impact on patients' quality of life, due to the progressive breathlessness, fatigue and physical limitations they entail. Although they affect the respiratory system, their causes, manifestations and management vary, making each disease unique in its evolution and treatment.

# 1. Idiopathic pulmonary fibrosis

**Idiopathic pulmonary fibrosis** (IPF) is a chronic, progressive lung disease characterized by the **abnormal development of scar tissue** (fibrosis) in the lungs. This fibrous tissue progressively replaces normal lung tissue, leading to **hardening of the alveolar walls**, preventing the lungs from expanding properly and facilitating gas exchange. Idiopathic pulmonary fibrosis is called "idiopathic" because its cause is unknown.

**Mechanism and pathophysiology**

In idiopathic pulmonary fibrosis, chronic inflammatory processes in the alveoli and interstitial lung tissue lead to the formation of **fibrosis**. This scar tissue prevents the lungs from functioning normally, reducing their capacity to expand and allow efficient gas exchange between blood and inspired air.

- **Thickening of lung tissue**: As fibrosis sets in, the lungs become rigid, making breathing difficult. Patients experience dyspnea (shortness of breath), often triggered by exertion, which worsens over time.

- **Decreased respiratory capacity**: as the disease progresses, the lungs' ability to transport oxygen in the

358

blood decreases, leading to **hypoxia** (lower oxygen levels in the blood) and a gradual decline in physical endurance.

## Symptoms

Patients with idiopathic pulmonary fibrosis have several symptoms, including:

- **Progressive dyspnea**: Shortness of breath is the most frequent symptom, becoming increasingly severe as fibrosis progresses. At first, it only appears with exertion, but over time it can occur even at rest.

- **Persistent dry cough**: A chronic cough, often non-productive (without sputum), is common in IPF.

- **Fatigue and weight loss**: Because breathing is difficult, patients may experience severe fatigue and involuntary weight loss.

## Diagnosis and treatment

**Diagnosis of** idiopathic pulmonary fibrosis is based on clinical examinations, **lung imaging** (such as high-resolution computed tomography), and sometimes lung biopsy. These examinations help identify areas of fibrosis in the lungs.

Treatment of IPF is primarily aimed at **slowing disease progression** and improving patients' quality of life, as there is currently no curative treatment.

- **Antifibrotic drugs**: Drugs such as pirfenidone and ninedanib are used to slow fibrosis progression.

- **Oxygen therapy**: When respiratory capacity is severely impaired, oxygen therapy may be necessary to compensate for hypoxia.

- **Lung transplantation**: In advanced cases, lung transplantation is sometimes considered as a treatment option.

## 2. Sarcoidosis

**Sarcoidosis** is a systemic inflammatory disease that can affect several organs, but mainly the **lungs and thoracic lymph nodes**. It is characterized by the formation of **granulomas**, clusters of inflammatory cells that disrupt the function of the organs they invade. Although the exact cause of sarcoidosis is unknown, it appears to result from an abnormal immune response triggered by environmental factors in genetically predisposed individuals.

**Mechanism and pathophysiology**

Sarcoidosis leads to the formation of **non-caseating granulomas**, abnormal cellular structures resulting from excessive activation of the immune system. These granulomas accumulate in the lungs, causing inflammation and disrupting gas exchange.

- **Lung inflammation**: in sarcoidosis, inflammation in the lungs can cause **thickening of the alveolar walls** and lead to fibrosis, reducing the lungs' ability to transport oxygen in the blood.

- **Multi-organ granulomas**: Although the lungs are mainly affected, sarcoidosis can affect other organs such as the skin, eyes, heart and nervous system, resulting in a wide variety of symptoms.

**Symptoms**

The symptoms of sarcoidosis vary according to the organs affected, but pulmonary manifestations are the most common.

- **Dry cough**: as in idiopathic pulmonary fibrosis, a **chronic cough** is common, accompanied by chest pain in some patients.

- **Shortness of breath**: **Dyspnea** may also occur, especially if granulomas affect large parts of the lungs.

- **Fatigue and fever**: Patients may also experience generalized fatigue and episodes of low-grade **fever**.

**Diagnosis and treatment**

**Diagnosis of** sarcoidosis is based on clinical examinations, **chest X-rays**, **CT scans** and **biopsies**, which confirm the presence of granulomas.

**Management of** sarcoidosis depends on the severity of the disease and the organs affected. In some patients, sarcoidosis may disappear on its own without treatment, while others require medical management.

- **Corticosteroids**: Corticosteroids (such as prednisone) are often used to reduce inflammation and control symptoms.

- **Immunosuppressants**: In more severe or chronic forms, immunosuppressants such as methotrexate or azathioprine may be prescribed.

- **Regular follow-up**: Careful monitoring is needed to track the progress of the disease, as it can recur or affect new organs.

# 3. Pulmonary hypertension

**Pulmonary hypertension** is a serious condition characterized by **increased blood pressure in the pulmonary arteries**, the vessels that carry blood from the heart to the lungs. This rise in pressure overloads the heart, particularly the **right ventricle**, which has to pump harder to send blood to the lungs. If left untreated, pulmonary hypertension can lead to **heart failure**.

## Mechanism and pathophysiology

Pulmonary hypertension can have many causes, but always involves **vasoconstriction** (narrowing) of the pulmonary arteries, **proliferation of** cells in the vascular wall, and sometimes the formation of **blood clots** that obstruct the pulmonary vessels. These mechanisms lead to increased resistance in the pulmonary arteries, forcing the heart to make an extra effort.

- **Right ventricular overload**: As the pressure in the lungs increases, the heart's **right ventricle** thickens (hypertrophies) and dilates, ultimately leading to **right heart failure**.

- **Decreased oxygenation**: due to malfunctioning pulmonary vessels, the blood is less well oxygenated, resulting in generalized **hypoxia**.

## Symptoms

Symptoms of pulmonary hypertension are often subtle at first, but become more marked as the disease progresses.

- **Shortness of breath**: as with pulmonary fibrosis and sarcoidosis, **dyspnea** is one of the main symptoms, particularly on exertion, but can also occur at rest in advanced stages.

- **Chest pain**: Patients may experience **chest pain** or a feeling of pressure in the heart.

- **Fatigue and edema**: Fatigue is a common symptom, sometimes accompanied by **edema** of the lower limbs (swelling of the feet and ankles), due to right heart failure.

**Diagnosis and treatment**

**Diagnosis** of pulmonary hypertension relies on imaging tests such as **echocardiography,** which measures pressure in the pulmonary arteries, and **functional tests** to assess exercise tolerance.

Treatment aims to **reduce pulmonary arterial pressure,** improve heart function and relieve symptoms.

- **Vasodilators:** drugs that dilate the pulmonary arteries, such as phosphodiesterase inhibitors (sildenafil) or prostacyclins, can be used to reduce vascular resistance.

- **Anticoagulants :** In cases where blood clots are present, anticoagulants may be prescribed to prevent complications.

- **Oxygen therapy and diuretics:** Oxygen therapy helps maintain adequate oxygen levels in the blood, while diuretics may be necessary to reduce edema.

  ◦ Management challenges in lesser-known pathologies

The management of **lesser-known pathologies** presents many challenges, both for patients and healthcare professionals. These diseases, often referred to as **rare** or under-studied **conditions,** include genetic, autoimmune, neurological and metabolic disorders. Their rarity and the complexity of their management, often compounded by a lack of medical knowledge, therapeutic resources and psychosocial support, make them particularly difficult to manage. These diseases are not only a medical challenge, but also an organizational, educational and emotional one, requiring close collaboration between patients, caregivers and specialists.

# 1. Diagnostic difficulties and delays in treatment

One of the main challenges of **rare or little-known pathologies** is **diagnosis**. Because of their rarity, these diseases are often poorly understood and difficult to identify, even for experienced professionals. This can lead to significant diagnostic delays, sometimes lasting several years, leaving patients in a state of uncertainty and suffering.

### Lack of knowledge and expertise

Rare pathologies are often poorly understood by the general public, but also by healthcare professionals. General practitioners and specialists may be unfamiliar with the atypical or specific symptoms of these diseases, which can lead to a series of **diagnostic errors** or consultations with numerous specialists before a precise diagnosis is made.

- **Complex differential diagnosis**: Rare diseases often share symptoms with more common conditions, making diagnosis difficult. Doctors have to rule out many other pathologies before thinking of a rare disease, which prolongs the diagnostic process.

- **Scarcity of specialized centers**: Only a few specialized medical centers or laboratories are equipped to carry out the tests needed to detect certain rare pathologies, and these centers are not always easily accessible to patients.

### Delayed care

Because of the difficulty of establishing a diagnosis, patients suffering from little-known pathologies may experience a **delay in** treatment, which worsens their state of health. This delay can have serious consequences, particularly if the disease progresses irreversibly without treatment.

- **Worsening of symptoms**: Patients may experience a worsening of their symptoms during the diagnosis phase, which can lead to complications, loss of autonomy, or a deterioration in their quality of life.

- **Frustration and emotional distress**: Uncertainty about the diagnosis generates **feelings of frustration and psychological distress** in patients and their families. They may feel misunderstood, abandoned by the healthcare system, and isolated in their journey.

## 2. Limitations of available treatments

Even after a precise diagnosis, the management of rare diseases is often complicated by the **lack of specific treatments**. Due to the low prevalence of these diseases, **pharmaceutical** and medical **research** is often less developed, and therapeutic options are limited or non-existent.

### Lack of specific treatments

Some rare diseases do not benefit from curative or effective treatments, as **clinical trials** are often rare or impossible to carry out, due to the small population affected. Available treatments are often aimed at relieving symptoms rather than treating the underlying cause of the disease.

- **Symptomatic therapies**: For many lesser-known pathologies, treatments focus on **managing symptoms** (pain, inflammation, fatigue) rather than curing them. This can maintain an acceptable quality of life, but does not stop the progression of the disease.

- **Non-adapted or off-label treatments**: In some cases, doctors have to prescribe "off-label" drugs, i.e. drugs designed for other pathologies, in the hope that they will have a beneficial effect on the rare disease. However, these treatments can carry the **risk of serious side effects**, as they have not been tested specifically for these conditions.

### Limited access to innovative therapies

**Innovative treatments**, such as **gene therapies** or **biologic therapies**, may represent an option for some patients with rare diseases. However, these treatments are often costly and not always available in all countries or health systems.

- **High treatment costs**: Drugs for rare diseases, often referred to as **"orphan drugs"**, can be extremely expensive. This can limit their accessibility, especially in healthcare systems where reimbursement is not guaranteed, leaving some patients without treatment.

- **Approval times**: Even if a new treatment is developed, there may be **significant delays** before it is approved or available in certain regions, prolonging the wait for patients.

# 3. Care coordination and multidisciplinary management

The management of rare diseases often requires a **multidisciplinary approach**, involving various specialists such as neurologists, pulmonologists, cardiologists, rheumatologists and geneticists. **Coordination of care** is therefore essential to provide comprehensive, coherent care, but it can be complicated to set up.

### Problem of fragmented care

One of the major challenges in the management of lesser-known pathologies is the **fragmentation of care**. Patients have to consult numerous specialists and undergo several examinations, sometimes in different institutions, which can make coherent management of their disease difficult.

- **Multiple players**: The patient may be followed by several specialists who do not always communicate effectively with each other, making it difficult to draw up a common care plan. There is a risk of **contradictory decisions** or **duplication of examinations**.

- **Role of the attending physician** : In many cases, the GP plays a central coordinating role, but may lack the specific expertise to manage the complex aspects of some rare diseases. **Fluid communication** between GPs and specialists is essential to ensure effective care.

**The need for personalized care**

Rare pathologies often require **personalized care**, adapted to the specific needs of each patient. This includes not only medical treatment, but also psychological support, physical rehabilitation and social accompaniment.

- **Individualized follow-up**: Each patient may present a different form of the disease, with varying progression and symptoms. It is therefore necessary to adapt treatment and care on a regular basis, according to the evolution of the patient's clinical condition.

- **Psychosocial support**: **Psychological** and social **support** is essential to help patients and their families cope with the emotional and practical consequences of illness. Social workers or psychologists specializing in chronic diseases may be needed to provide advice, resources and guidance.

## 4. Patient isolation and lack of support

Another often overlooked aspect of rare or little-known diseases is the **isolation** felt by patients and their families. The lack of knowledge and awareness around these diseases can make the medical and personal journey extremely difficult, both in terms of access to information and community support.

**Social and emotional isolation**

Suffering from a rare disease can lead to considerable **social isolation**. Patients and their families can feel misunderstood by those around them, and often helpless in the face of a disease that few people, even within the medical community, know the ins and outs of.

- **Stigmatization and misunderstanding**: The invisibility of certain rare diseases can lead to misunderstanding on the part of family and friends, who don't always perceive the extent of the difficulties encountered by the patient. This can lead to feelings of **loneliness** and **stigmatization**.

- **Depression and anxiety**: The stress of uncertain diagnosis, disease progression and lack of treatment options can exacerbate **mental health** problems such as depression and anxiety.

**Lack of structural support**

Rare disease patients may also encounter a **lack of structural support**, both within the healthcare system and from **patient networks**. The absence of dedicated support groups or adapted resources often complicates their search for information and help.

- **Patient organizations**: Some rare disease **associations** or **support groups** exist, but they are not always well developed or accessible. These structures can offer valuable support in terms of information sharing, practical resources and moral support.

- **Lack of awareness**: There is often a **lack of awareness of rare diseases** in society in general, including among healthcare professionals, which complicates the search for appropriate solutions for the day-to-day management of the disease.

- **Special care for patients with rare respiratory diseases**
  - ○ Monitoring and managing complex symptoms

**Monitoring and managing complex symptoms** are essential elements in the management of patients suffering from chronic, multi-systemic or advanced diseases. These symptoms, often multiple and interdependent, require constant attention and a multidisciplinary approach to minimize the impact on the patient's quality of life. Managing complex symptoms requires not only clinical expertise, but also the ability to adapt care on an individual basis, taking into account disease progression, ongoing treatments and the patient's overall well-being.

# 1. Understanding the complexity of symptoms

**Complex symptoms** are characterized by their intensity, persistence and tendency to affect several aspects of the patient's life. They may be linked to a primary disease, or be the result of co-morbidities and treatments. Chronic pain, shortness of breath, fatigue, cognitive impairment, nausea or depressive symptoms are all manifestations which, when they coexist, make management more difficult.

### Multifactorial nature of symptoms

Complex symptoms are often **multifactorial in** nature, meaning they result from several simultaneous causes. For example, a patient with advanced cancer may suffer from neuropathic pain linked to the tumor, fatigue due to chemotherapy, and shortness of breath due to a pulmonary complication. This interaction between different symptoms worsens the patient's overall situation.

- **Pain**: Pain can be inflammatory, mechanical, neuropathic or mixed. It can affect various parts of the body, and requires different treatments depending on its cause and intensity.

- **Fatigue**: Chronic fatigue is often difficult to assess and may be linked to the disease itself, to treatment or to

369

psychological factors. It is frequently accompanied by loss of motivation and sleep disorders.

- **Shortness of breath (dyspnea)**: In respiratory pathologies such as COPD or heart failure, breathlessness is a complex symptom that impacts mobility and leads to a feeling of anxiety, worsening the patient's condition.

**Interaction between symptoms**

One of the characteristics of complex symptoms is their **interaction**. One symptom may aggravate another, creating a vicious circle. For example, a patient suffering from chronic pain may have trouble sleeping, which worsens fatigue and perceived pain. Similarly, anxiety can amplify dyspnea, leading to increased fatigue.

- **Domino effect**: For example, **poorly controlled pain** can lead to appetite problems, weight loss and general weakness, which in turn aggravate pain and other symptoms such as insomnia or depression.

## 2. Monitoring complex symptoms

**Monitoring** complex symptoms is essential to assess their evolution, adjust treatments in real time and prevent complications. This requires careful clinical observation, the use of appropriate measuring tools, and constant communication between the patient and the care team.

**Continuous clinical monitoring**

**Regular clinical monitoring** enables early identification of changes in the patient's condition, particularly in the event of deterioration. This includes assessment of pain, breathing, vital functions, mental state and nutrition.

- **Pain measurement**: **Pain scales** (such as the visual analog scale or the numerical scale) can be used to assess pain intensity at different times of the day. Regular pain assessment helps to adjust analgesic doses and choose appropriate treatments (analgesics, opioids, anti-inflammatories, etc.).

- **Vital parameters**: Monitoring vital constants (respiratory rate, blood pressure, heart rate, oxygen saturation) is crucial for patients with respiratory or cardiovascular diseases. These parameters enable early detection of decompensation and rapid adjustment of treatments.

- **Psychological follow-up**: It's also important to regularly assess the patient's **mental state**, especially for those suffering from complex symptoms linked to chronic pathologies. Stress, anxiety and depression are often under-diagnosed, even though they have a considerable impact on the perception and intensity of other symptoms.

## Monitoring tools

To facilitate **ongoing monitoring**, various tools and technologies are available to help track the evolution of symptoms in real time.

- **Telemonitoring**: Telemonitoring systems enable patients to measure their oxygen saturation, heart rate or blood pressure at home, with results sent directly to the medical team. This is particularly useful for patients suffering from heart or respiratory failure.

- **Diaries**: **Symptom diaries**, in which patients note the intensity of their pain, their fatigue or their emotions, give caregivers a precise overview of the daily evolution of symptoms, enabling them to better adapt treatments.

# 3. Managing complex symptoms

The **management of** complex symptoms is based on a **multidimensional** approach, in which several therapeutic modalities are combined to relieve symptoms while improving the patient's overall comfort. This approach includes medical treatments, palliative care, psychological interventions and lifestyle adjustments.

## Medication management

One of the first steps in managing complex symptoms is to adjust **medication regimens**. Medications are used to reduce pain, relieve fatigue, manage dyspnea, or treat the side effects of the treatments themselves.

- **Pain medication: analgesics**, whether simple (paracetamol) or more powerful (opioids), are adjusted according to the nature and intensity of the pain. It is also common to use co-analgesics, such as antidepressants or anticonvulsants, to treat neuropathic pain.

- **Treating fatigue: Chronic fatigue** is difficult to treat directly. However, by improving sleep (with medication or behavioral therapies) and treating underlying causes (anemia, malnutrition), we can often improve the patient's quality of life.

- **Treatment of respiratory disorders**: For patients suffering from dyspnea, **bronchodilators**, **steroids** or **diuretics** may be required, depending on the cause of the dyspnea. In severe cases, **oxygen therapy** or **non-invasive ventilation** may be used.

## Non-pharmacological approaches

As a complement to drug treatments, **non-pharmacological approaches** play a key role in the management of complex symptoms. These interventions can help improve pain tolerance, reduce stress and promote better adaptation to symptoms.

- **Physiotherapy and rehabilitation**: **Physiotherapy** is often used to maintain mobility, reduce pain and improve respiratory capacity. For patients with complex respiratory symptoms, controlled breathing exercises or physiotherapy techniques can help relieve dyspnea.

- **Relaxation techniques and stress management**: **Relaxation techniques** such as meditation, deep breathing or progressive muscle relaxation are very useful for patients with complex symptoms. They help reduce anxiety, which can exacerbate the perception of pain and shortness of breath.

- **Behavioral therapy and psychological support**: **Psychological support** is essential to help patients cope with complex symptoms. Cognitive-behavioural therapies (CBT) can help to modify pain perception and develop strategies for living better with fatigue or breathlessness.

### Multidisciplinary approach

Managing complex symptoms requires a **multidisciplinary approach** involving a variety of specialists, such as doctors, nurses, physiotherapists, psychologists and sometimes social workers. This collaboration enables all aspects of the disease to be covered, and care to be tailored to the patient's individual needs.

- **Care coordination**: Coordination between the various care providers is essential to ensure smooth, coherent care. Patients benefit from harmonized care, avoiding fragmented interventions.

- **Personalized care plan**: Each patient must have a **personalized care plan**, regularly re-evaluated, which takes into account the evolution of symptoms and the impact of treatments. This plan includes both medical (symptom relief) and quality-of-life objectives.

       ◦   Teamwork with specialists for adapted care protocols

**Teamwork with specialists** to establish and apply **appropriate care protocols** is a fundamental element in patient management, especially when dealing with complex or chronic pathologies. A multidisciplinary approach is essential to holistic care, as it brings together the expertise of several healthcare professionals to address the various aspects of the disease. By working together, medical specialists, nurses, physiotherapists, caregivers and other members of the care team can develop **personalized care protocols** optimized for each patient. These protocols help to improve the quality of care, ensure continuity of intervention and prevent potential complications.

# 1. The need for a multidisciplinary approach

**Complex chronic diseases**, such as diabetes, pulmonary pathologies (like COPD or severe asthma), cancers or neurodegenerative diseases, often require comprehensive and prolonged care. In these contexts, a single discipline is not sufficient to meet all the patient's needs, as these diseases affect several body systems and impact on physical, mental and social health.

**Complementary expertise**

Each specialist brings a **unique expertise** to the patient's care, contributing to a more comprehensive assessment of the patient's condition and the development of more effective solutions.

- **General practitioner**: The general practitioner is often the **main coordinator of** care. They ensure continuity of care, manage day-to-day symptoms and refer patients to specialists according to their specific needs. They play a crucial role in linking specialists with the patient.

- **Specialist physicians: Cardiologists, pulmonologists, oncologists, neurologists** and other specialists bring their targeted expertise to bear on the patient's specific pathologies. They prescribe treatments, monitor their effectiveness and adjust protocols as the disease progresses.

- **Nurses: Nurses** are often the team members who spend the most time with patients. They play a key role in monitoring clinical signs, administering treatment and communicating with other healthcare professionals. They also ensure coordination between specialists, and can quickly report any changes in the patient's condition.

- **Physiotherapists and rehabilitators: Physiotherapists** or **physiotherapists** intervene to help maintain or restore mobility, manage pain and strengthen physical capacities. In the case of respiratory illnesses, for example, they teach breathing techniques or encourage the expectoration of bronchial secretions.

**A holistic view of the patient**

Collaboration between different specialists ensures a **holistic view of** the patient. Instead of focusing solely on a specific disease or symptom, the multidisciplinary approach takes into account all aspects of the patient's health. This holistic approach helps to **anticipate complications**, avoid undesirable treatment effects and adapt care to the patient's tolerance and needs.

## 2. Implementation of personalized care protocols

The creation of **appropriate care protocols** is a central element of multidisciplinary teamwork. These protocols are **detailed plans** that define the stages of care, the treatments to be followed, and the roles of each person involved. They ensure **consistency of** care and enable us to respond to the specific needs of each patient.

### Initial assessment and definition of objectives

The first step in developing an appropriate care protocol is a thorough **initial assessment of** the patient. This assessment includes not only medical aspects, but also psychological, social and functional dimensions.

- **Diagnosis and clinical evaluation**: The team assesses the patient's general state of health through clinical examinations, imaging, laboratory analyses and specialized consultations. This stage is crucial to understanding the pathology and its evolution.

- **Defining therapeutic objectives**: Following this assessment, **therapeutic objectives** are defined. These goals may be curative, in the case of treatable diseases, or palliative, when the aim is to improve quality of life and manage symptoms in chronic or terminal illnesses. The team must ensure that these goals are realistic and focused on the patient's well-being.

### Collaboration on protocol development

Once the objectives have been set, each specialist contributes to the care protocol, making recommendations based on his or her expertise. For example:

- **Drug treatments**: The specialist prescribes treatments specific to the pathology (chemotherapy for cancer, antibiotics for a lung infection, etc.). The pharmacist can also intervene to ensure that there are no interactions between drugs, and to adjust dosages.

- **Functional rehabilitation**: Physiotherapists can recommend **functional rehabilitation** sessions to prevent loss of mobility or improve respiratory capacity, in the case of lung or neuromuscular diseases.

- **Psychological support**: A **psychologist** or **psychiatrist** can be integrated into the team if the patient shows signs of depression, anxiety or emotional distress linked to their illness or treatment.

### Protocol adaptation and monitoring

Care protocols are not set in stone: they need to be constantly **adapted** to the patient's response to treatment and to the evolution of the disease. Communication between team members is crucial to ensure that the care plan remains relevant and optimal.

- **Team meetings**: Regular meetings between specialists enable them to review the patient's condition, discuss the effectiveness of current treatments and suggest adjustments. These meetings also enable interventions to be coordinated to avoid redundancies or contradictions in care.

- **Continuous monitoring**: The protocol often includes elements of **clinical monitoring**, such as regular measurement of vital parameters (heart rate, blood pressure, oxygen saturation) or biological tests to check tolerance to treatment.

## 3. Team coordination and communication

**Fluid communication** between the different team members is essential to ensure coherent, effective care. Each healthcare professional must be informed of the others' interventions, to ensure that all actions are aligned and adapted to the patient's needs.

**Use of communication tools**

The use of appropriate **communication tools** facilitates the sharing of information between the various professionals involved in patient care.

- **Shared medical record**: A **shared electronic medical record** enables all healthcare professionals to access a patient's medical information in real time. This makes it possible to avoid redundancies, monitor disease progression and ensure traceability of medical decisions.

- **Care booklet**: A **care booklet** can also be given to the patient or family. This booklet contains essential information on the treatment plan, prescribed medication, appointments and important instructions.

**Continuing education and interprofessional collaboration**

Managing patients with complex pathologies requires team members to be well-trained in the latest techniques and protocols. **Ongoing training** and **inter-professional exchanges** are therefore essential to maintaining a high level of competence and integrating the latest innovations into clinical practice.

- **Interdisciplinary seminars**: Seminars or training courses bringing together healthcare professionals from different disciplines enable them to share knowledge and experience in the management of complex diseases.

- **Regular exchanges**: **Collaboration** should be encouraged by creating opportunities for formal and informal exchanges between team members. These exchanges enable practical problems to be resolved quickly, and improve the quality of care.

# 4. Involving the patient in the care protocol

It is essential to **involve the patient** in the creation and implementation of his or her care protocol. The patient must be considered a **central player** in his or her treatment, being informed and consulted at every stage of the process.

**Information sharing**

Healthcare professionals must ensure that the patient understands the **goals of treatment**, the options available, and the risks and benefits of each approach.

- **Clear, transparent information**: Explanations must be adapted to the patient's level of understanding, and delivered in a clear and caring manner. The patient must feel confident enough to ask questions and express concerns.

- **Informed consent**: Before implementing a complex treatment or protocol, the patient's informed consent is required. This implies that the patient is fully aware of what is at stake and can actively participate in the decision-making process.

**Empowerment and support**

Encouraging patients to take **charge** of their **own** care helps them to better manage the chronic aspects of their disease. This involves learning simple therapeutic gestures, such as self-monitoring of symptoms (for example, measuring blood sugar levels for a diabetic patient) or self-administration of certain treatments.

- **Therapeutic education**: **Therapeutic education** is an invaluable tool for helping patients to better understand their disease, current treatments and the actions they need to adopt on a daily basis. A well-informed patient is more likely to follow medical recommendations and report any abnormalities promptly.


- **Emotional and psychological support for rare diseases**
  - Helping patients and families manage difficult diagnoses

Helping patients and their families cope with a **difficult diagnosis** is a delicate task, requiring not only medical skills, but also an empathetic approach, active listening and ongoing psychological support. Difficult diagnoses can involve serious, chronic, progressive or incurable illnesses, such as cancer, neurodegenerative diseases, or certain rare genetic conditions. When these diagnoses are made, patients and their families are often faced with a complex set of emotions, ranging from initial shock through fear, worry and emotional distress to gradual acceptance. Multidimensional support is essential to help them navigate this difficult period and adapt to the new reality.

# 1. Announcing the diagnosis: managing the initial shock

The **announcement of a diagnosis** is often a moment of great emotional intensity. It marks the beginning of a long road for the patient and his or her loved ones. The way in which this information is communicated plays a decisive role in how patients and their families cope with the situation. The announcement must therefore be made with great sensitivity, while ensuring that the information provided is clear and adapted to the patient's capacity to assimilate it.

### Creating an environment conducive to listening

When a difficult diagnosis is announced, it's vital to create a **calm, supportive environment** where patients and their families feel safe and confident.

- **Emotional availability**: It's important for the doctor or healthcare professional to be fully present, without being pressed for time. The patient must have the opportunity to ask questions, express fears and reflect on what has just been announced.

- **Appropriate language**: Complex medical terms need to be explained in a way that patients and their families can understand. Using **simple language**, without minimizing the seriousness of the diagnosis, helps to avoid confusion or misinterpretation.

### Managing immediate emotions

**Shock**, **disbelief** and **denial** are common emotional reactions to the news of a difficult diagnosis. The healthcare professional's role is to help the patient and family **digest the information**, while supporting them through this initial emotional stage.

- **Active listening**: It's essential to welcome emotions with kindness and without judgment. Active listening allows us to recognize feelings of anger, sadness or dismay, while providing a safe space for these emotions to express themselves.

- **Answering immediate questions**: Although the initial state of shock can make it difficult to understand all the details of the diagnosis, it's important to answer immediate questions and clarify the most urgent practical or medical aspects.

## 2. Emotional support: helping to understand and accept

After the diagnosis, patients and their families face an **emotional reorganization**. Acceptance of the diagnosis can take time, and caregivers need to offer **empathic support throughout** this adjustment phase. This accompaniment includes emotional support, but also access to resources and information to better understand the disease and the stages to come.

**Encouraging emotional expression**

It is essential to encourage patients and their families to **express their emotions**, rather than repressing them. Acceptance of the diagnosis means not only understanding the seriousness of the disease, but also accepting it emotionally.

- **Psychological support**: Offering consultations with a **psychologist** or **psychiatrist** specialized in supporting patients with serious illnesses can be beneficial. These professionals help manage the intense emotions such as anxiety, depression or anger that can arise after a difficult diagnosis.

- **Support groups**: Joining **support groups** enables patients and their families to share their experiences with others in similar situations. This form of support encourages the expression of emotions and helps break the isolation often felt after a serious diagnosis.

**Provide clear, understandable information**

Uncertainty is one of the greatest sources of stress for patients and their loved ones following a difficult diagnosis. They need **understanding and clarity** to know what lies ahead, what to expect in terms of disease progression, and what treatments are available.

- **Explaining treatment options**: Providing detailed information on treatment options helps patients to feel more involved in their care. This helps them regain some **control** over their situation, despite the severity of the disease.

- **Written documentation**: It can be useful to provide patients and their families with **brochures** or **documents explaining** the disease, its treatments, and the palliative or supportive care available. This enables them to reread the information afterwards and gain a better understanding at their own pace.

## 3. Decision-making support: providing a framework for informed choice

Another crucial aspect of managing a difficult diagnosis is **making decisions** about treatment, organization of care and sometimes **palliative care**. Patients and their families are often faced with complex and emotionally challenging decisions, such as choosing between treatment options with uncertain outcomes, or discussing end-of-life wishes.

**Helping you make informed choices**

Healthcare professionals play a central role in enabling patients to make informed decisions, by providing clear, comprehensive and objective information on the benefits and risks of different treatments.

- **Explanation of benefits and risks**: Each therapeutic option should be explained in simple terms, highlighting the potential benefits and associated risks. This enables patients to **weigh up the pros and cons, and** make choices that reflect their priorities and values.

- **Decision support**: **Decision support** involves accompanying patients and their loved ones in their reflections. This process includes listening carefully to their concerns and preferences, and taking these into account in the development of the care plan.

### Respecting patient autonomy

Respecting patients' **autonomy** is a key principle when dealing with difficult diagnoses. Even in the face of serious illness, it is essential that patients retain the ability to **choose** how they wish to approach their illness and its treatment.

- **Informed consent**: All treatment must be offered with the patient's **informed consent**. This means that the patient fully understands what each treatment entails, including palliative care, and can freely choose or refuse the proposed options.

- **Family support**: It's also crucial to support families in this decision-making process, especially when the patient is no longer able to make decisions for themselves. They must be guided in respecting the patient's wishes, while helping them to cope with their own emotions and responsibilities.

## 4. Long-term care: ongoing support and palliative care

**Difficult diagnoses** often require **long-term management**, during which the patient and family will need ongoing support. Treatment and symptom management, as well as psychological and emotional follow-up, need to be integrated into a coherent overall approach, with regular adaptation of care as the disease progresses.

### Palliative care and quality of life

In certain advanced or incurable illnesses, **palliative care** becomes an essential part of support. This care aims to improve the patient's **quality of life** by relieving pain and other symptoms, rather than attempting to cure the disease.

- **Symptom management**: Palliative care includes managing **pain**, shortness of breath, fatigue and other physical symptoms that can become overwhelming as the disease progresses. The goal is to make the last months or years of life as comfortable as possible.

- **Psychological and spiritual support**: Palliative care also includes psychological and sometimes spiritual support, to help patients and their families cope with the imminence of death, manage complex emotions and find meaning at this stage of life.

**Support for caregivers**

**Family carers** play a central role in supporting patients coping with serious illnesses. However, their emotional and physical burden is often immense, and they too need support.

- **Support for caregivers**: It is essential to provide **specific support** for caregivers, by training them in care techniques, offering them periods of respite, and making psychological support resources available to them.

- **Preventing burnout**: Caregiver burnout can be detrimental to the well-being of both the caregiver and the patient. It is therefore important to offer them time to rest, as well as social and medical support, so that they can continue to help their loved one without feeling overwhelmed.

  - The importance of empathetic listening and personalized support

The **importance of empathetic listening** and **personalized support** in healthcare cannot be underestimated. These elements form the basis of a trusting relationship between caregiver and patient, and have a direct impact on the quality of care provided, patient satisfaction and clinical outcomes. Empathic listening and personalized support go far beyond simple observation or the administration of treatments: they encompass a deep understanding of the patient's emotional, physical and psychological needs, with the aim of providing holistic, individualized care. This approach is particularly crucial in situations where the patient is faced with serious, chronic or complex illnesses, and where emotional support and trust in the healthcare team are essential to better cope with the disease and adhere to treatment.

## 1. Empathic listening: an essential foundation in the caregiver-patient relationship

**Empathic listening** is a key skill in caregiver-patient communication. It involves paying sympathetic attention to what the patient is saying, to his or her emotions, fears and expectations, without judgment or interruption. This form of listening goes beyond words; it also involves picking up **non-verbal cues**, such as body language, facial expressions and tone of voice, to fully understand what the patient is feeling.

### Developing a relationship of trust

Empathic listening creates a **bond of trust** between patient and caregiver. When patients feel genuinely listened to, they are more inclined to express their fears, doubts and concerns. This climate of trust is particularly crucial in vulnerable situations, such as the announcement of a serious diagnosis or during complex treatment.

- **Reduced anxiety**: By making patients feel understood, empathic listening helps reduce **anxiety** and uncertainty. The simple fact of being heard and taken seriously helps to alleviate feelings of stress, especially at times when patients feel helpless in the face of their illness.

- **Facilitating dialogue**: Empathic listening encourages **open** and honest **dialogue**. When the patient feels that the caregiver is fully engaged in the conversation, he or she is more likely to ask questions, clarify doubts, or talk about symptoms or details that might otherwise be overlooked.

**Understanding people beyond their symptoms**

Empathy involves **seeing the person behind the patient**, understanding his or her life context, values, fears and desires. A caregiver who listens with empathy doesn't focus solely on medical symptoms, but seeks to understand what's important to the whole person.

- **Taking emotional and social factors into account**: For example, a patient may not adhere to a treatment not because they don't want to, but because psychosocial factors, such as fear of losing their job or family responsibilities, prevent them from doing so. Empathic listening helps to uncover these aspects and respond appropriately.

- **Recognizing emotional needs**: Empathy also enables us to recognize the **emotional needs** that often accompany illness. These may include fear of death, social isolation, or the emotional pain associated with loss of autonomy. By understanding these emotions, caregivers can adjust their approach to offer not only physical care, but also psychological support.

# 2. Personalized support: care tailored to each patient's specific needs

**Personalized care** goes hand in hand with empathetic listening. It's an approach that aims to provide care tailored to each patient's individual needs, taking into account not only their physical condition, but also their preferences, beliefs and environment. Unlike a standardized approach, which may not be suitable for everyone, personalized care seeks to individualize every aspect of care.

**Adapting treatments to patient preferences**

Every patient is unique, and his or her relationship to illness, treatment and health in general differs. **Personalized support** enables care and treatment to be tailored to the patient's preferences.

- **Respect for patient choice**: For example, some patients may prefer to limit medical interventions in favor of a better quality of life, while others will choose to undergo more aggressive treatments to prolong their survival. **Respecting** patients' **choices** and values is a fundamental aspect of personalized care.

- **Taking cultural and religious beliefs into account**: Personal beliefs, whether cultural or religious, often play a role in how patients want to be treated. For example, a patient may refuse certain treatments because of his or her spiritual beliefs. Personalized support allows us to respect these beliefs while seeking alternatives that meet the patient's medical needs.

**Individualizing care to meet changing needs**

A patient's needs evolve throughout the course of their care. **Personalized support** adapts to changes in health status, new emotional realities and changing patient priorities.

- **Regular re-evaluation**: A personalized care plan must be **re-evaluated regularly** to ensure that it continues to meet the patient's needs. If a patient with a chronic illness deteriorates, it may be necessary to modify treatments or introduce palliative care.

- **Listening to patient feedback**: Personalized support also means taking into account **patients' feedback** on their treatments. A drug may be effective from a medical point of view, but cause side effects that are too much for the patient to bear. Adapting treatment to the patient's feelings is an integral part of this approach.

## 3. Positive impact of empathetic listening and personalized support

**Empathetic listening** and **personalized support** bring many benefits for patients and caregivers alike. They help create a more **humanized** care environment, where patients feel they are cared for holistically and not just medically.

### Improving the quality of care

When care is personalized and based on empathic listening, the **quality of care** improves considerably. The patient feels more involved in his or her own treatment, and this in turn promotes **adherence**.

- **Increased compliance**: Patients who feel listened to and whose needs are taken into account are more likely to follow medical recommendations, as they better understand the aims of treatment and feel involved in decisions concerning their health.

- **Preventing complications**: Empathetic listening enables **early detection of** signs of complications or deteriorating health. By being attentive to what the patient is expressing, the caregiver can intervene more quickly and adjust treatments, thereby reducing the risk of serious complications.

**Emotional support and overall well-being**

Personalized care also offers valuable **emotional support** to patients and their families, taking into account their emotions and psychological needs. This helps to improve patients' overall well-being, even in difficult medical situations.

- **Reduced stress and anxiety**: Simply knowing that you are understood and cared for holistically can significantly reduce the **stress** and **anxiety** associated with illness. This makes it easier to manage symptoms and treatment.

- **Improved quality of life**: By adapting care to the patient's priorities and providing emotional support, we help to improve overall **quality of life**, despite the severity of the disease.

# 4. Involving families in personalized support

Personalized support is not limited to the patient alone, but often includes the **involvement of families in** the care process. The patient's loved ones play an essential role, both in providing emotional support and in the day-to-day management of the disease.

**Supporting caregivers**

**Family caregivers** also need personalized support, as they are often on the front line in supporting the patient. They can carry a heavy emotional and physical burden, and need to be supported in this role.

- **Psychological support**: Offering caregivers **psychological support** helps prevent emotional exhaustion and helps them cope with the challenges of caring for a sick loved one.

- **Practical training**: In certain situations, families need to be trained in homecare **techniques** or treatment administration. Personalized support for caregivers helps them to feel competent and to manage the patient's day-to-day care with greater confidence.

## Taking family dynamics into account

Empathetic listening and personalized support also take **family dynamics** into account. Caregivers need to be sensitive to interactions and potential tensions within the family, particularly in situations of serious illness or at the end of life.

- **Conflict management**: It may be necessary to intervene to **manage conflict** or disagreement within the family regarding medical decisions. By listening and understanding everyone's point of view, the caregiver can facilitate decision-making and maintain a harmonious environment.

# Chapter 14

# Care for patients with respiratory disabilities

- **Understanding the specific needs of disabled patients**
  - Motor, neuromuscular or congenital disabilities affecting breathing

**Motor, neuromuscular or congenital disabilities** that affect breathing present complex challenges for patients and carers alike. These conditions can seriously compromise respiratory function by impacting the muscles responsible for breathing, or by limiting thoracic mobility, leading to difficulties in breathing correctly and maintaining good oxygenation. Managing these pathologies requires a comprehensive approach, tailored to each individual, combining medical treatment, rehabilitation, respiratory assistance and psychosocial support.

# 1. The different causes of disabilities affecting breathing

**Motor**, **neuromuscular** or **congenital disabilities** that affect breathing encompass several types of condition, each with a specific impact on the respiratory system. These pathologies alter the patient's ability to **control the respiratory muscles**, maintain efficient breathing or mobilize sufficient air in the lungs.

**Neuromuscular pathologies**

Neuromuscular diseases affect the **nerves** and **muscles** that control breathing, leading to progressive muscle weakness. Among the most common:

- **Duchenne muscular dystrophy**: This hereditary disease causes **progressive degeneration of muscles**, including those responsible for breathing. As the muscles weaken, the ability of the lungs to inflate and empty is reduced, leading to advanced respiratory failure.

- **Amyotrophic lateral sclerosis (ALS)**: ALS affects **motor neurons**, leading to progressive paralysis of voluntary muscles, including those involved in breathing. In advanced stages, atrophy of the intercostal muscles and

394

diaphragm prevents autonomous breathing, necessitating the use of assisted ventilation.

- **Myasthenia gravis**: This autoimmune disease causes **excessive fatigue of the muscles**, including the respiratory muscles. Episodes of muscle weakness can cause sudden breathing difficulties, requiring monitoring and respiratory support.

## Motor disabilities

Certain non-neuromuscular **motor disabilities**, such as spinal cord trauma or congenital malformations, can also affect breathing by limiting thoracic mobility or paralyzing the respiratory muscles.

- **Spinal cord injury**: Damage to the spinal cord, particularly at the cervical level, can lead to **paralysis of the intercostal muscles and diaphragm**, considerably reducing the ability to breathe independently.

- **Rett syndrome**: This rare genetic disorder mainly affects girls and causes motor development disorders, leading to intermittent breathing difficulties due to a **neurological dysfunction** affecting respiration.

## Congenital malformations

Some **congenital malformations** have a direct impact on the respiratory system, either by limiting normal lung growth or by affecting the muscles required for breathing.

- **Spina bifida**: When this congenital malformation affects the spinal cord, it can lead to **partial or complete paralysis of** the muscles required for breathing, particularly in cases of high spina bifida.

- **Narrow rib cage syndrome**: This syndrome affects the bony structure of the thorax, reducing the space available for the lungs. This limits the ability of the lungs to inflate fully, leading to chronic hypoventilation.

## 2. Impact on respiratory function

The **respiratory problems** associated with these disabilities can be varied, ranging from mild difficulty in breathing to complete inability to maintain adequate ventilation without assistance. The main effects observed include respiratory muscle weakness, hypoventilation, frequent respiratory infections and impaired secretion management.

### Respiratory muscle weakness

**Weak respiratory muscles** prevent efficient ventilation. Patients may find it difficult to inhale enough air (restrictive ventilatory insufficiency) or to exhale properly, leading to an **accumulation of carbon dioxide** in the blood (hypercapnia).

- **Reduced vital capacity**: Total lung capacity is reduced, as the muscles responsible for thoracic expansion (diaphragm, intercostals) are weakened. This leads to reduced gas exchange, resulting in **hypoxemia** (lack of oxygen in the blood).

- **Nocturnal respiratory disorders**: Patients may suffer from **alveolar hypoventilation syndrome**, particularly during sleep, when breathing is less consciously controlled. This leads to frequent awakenings, morning headaches and daytime sleepiness.

### Secretion management

**Impaired coughing** is frequently observed in these pathologies, as coughing requires strong contraction of the abdominal and intercostal muscles to expel secretions from the respiratory tract.

- **Accumulation of secretions**: The inability to properly evacuate bronchial secretions can lead to **recurrent respiratory infections**, such as bronchitis or pneumonia. Stagnant secretions can also lead to airway obstruction.

- **Superinfections**: The risk of **pulmonary superinfections** increases in these patients due to the accumulation of mucus in the respiratory tract. Specific measures, such as the use of cough-assist devices, are often required.

## 3. Medical management and respiratory support

The management of **motor, neuromuscular or congenital disabilities** affecting breathing requires a multidisciplinary approach integrating **medical treatments, specific respiratory interventions, rehabilitation** and **technological support** to ensure adequate ventilation and maintain optimum quality of life.

### Assisted ventilation and oxygen therapy

In the most severe cases, **ventilatory assistance** is often required to compensate for respiratory muscle weakness and ensure an adequate supply of oxygen.

- **Non-invasive ventilation (NIV)**: NIV is often used in patients suffering from nocturnal hypoventilation or moderate muscle weakness. It can be applied via a **nasal** or face **mask** during the night, relieving the load on respiratory muscles and preventing hypoventilation.

- **Invasive ventilation**: In patients who have lost the ability to breathe independently, **tracheostomy** and mechanical ventilation are sometimes required to maintain ventilation. These devices provide continuous respiratory assistance.

- **Oxygen therapy**: In situations where hypoxia is present despite adequate ventilation, **oxygen therapy** can be used to increase the concentration of inspired oxygen and improve the patient's oxygen saturation.

**Respiratory physiotherapy**

**Respiratory rehabilitation** plays a key role in maintaining respiratory muscles and managing secretions. It includes specific exercises to strengthen respiratory capacity and techniques to improve secretion evacuation.

- **Breathing exercises**: Physiotherapists can teach **breathing exercises** to strengthen the diaphragm and improve respiratory coordination. Techniques such as **diaphragmatic breathing and** inspiratory muscle strengthening exercises help maximize remaining respiratory function.

- **De-clogging techniques**: Devices such as **cough-assist** or **chest percussion** can be used to help patients expel secretions, preventing bronchial congestion and reducing the risk of infection.

**Multidisciplinary follow-up and palliative care**

Effective management of respiratory disability requires a **multidisciplinary approach** involving general practitioners, pulmonologists, neurologists, physiotherapists, occupational therapists and palliative care teams.

- **Coordinated care**: Regular follow-up by a **pulmonologist** is essential to adjust ventilation requirements and monitor respiratory function. In addition, collaboration with **nutritionists** may be necessary to adapt the diet, as appropriate nutrition is crucial to sustain muscle strength.

- **Palliative care**: In cases where the disease is progressive and active management can no longer maintain respiratory function satisfactorily, **palliative care** plays a key role. It aims to ensure patient comfort, relieve symptoms and improve quality of life.

# 4. Psychosocial support and improved quality of life

Living with a **breathing disability** brings not only physical challenges, but also significant psychological and social consequences. Feelings of dependence, physical limitations and uncertainty about the course of the disease can lead to anxiety, depression and social isolation.

**Psychological support**

**Psychological support** is crucial to help patients cope with the emotional challenges associated with their condition. Patients may need support to accept their loss of autonomy, adapt to the use of respiratory equipment and manage uncertainties about their prognosis.

- **Managing anxiety**: **Anxiety** is common in patients with respiratory disorders, particularly in cases of severe dyspnea. Relaxation techniques, such as **meditation** or **controlled breathing**, can help relieve anxiety and improve tolerance to episodes of respiratory distress.

- **Support groups**: Participation in **support groups** where patients share their experiences can also be beneficial. This helps to create a support network and combat isolation.

**Home adaptations**

Improving the **quality of life** of patients with respiratory disabilities also requires **adaptations to the home** to make daily life easier.

- **Home medical equipment**: The installation of devices such as ventilators, oxygen therapy or respiratory decluttering equipment must be designed to make them as easy and effective to use as possible in the home environment.

- **Technical aids**: Occupational therapists can provide **technical aids** to help with everyday tasks, such as transfers or managing activities of daily living.

  ◦  Adapting management to provide optimal care

**Adapting care to deliver optimal results** is an essential approach in the medical field, particularly when dealing with complex, chronic or progressive pathologies. This adaptation relies on the ability of healthcare professionals to constantly adjust care to the patient's evolving state of health, specific needs and personal preferences. The aim is not to apply standardized treatments, but to adopt an individualized approach that takes into account the physical, psychological and social changes of each patient. This flexibility in treatment not only improves the effectiveness of care, but also optimizes the patient's quality of life throughout his or her healthcare journey.

# 1. Understanding the specific needs of each patient

The first step in adapting care is to **understand the specific needs** of each patient. Each individual is unique, with medical histories, psychological factors, expectations and social constraints all influencing the way the disease is experienced and managed. It is therefore crucial to adopt a holistic approach that goes beyond simple clinical management, taking into account **physical, emotional and social** aspects.

**Consideration of physical and medical factors**

The patient's **medical profile**, including underlying pathologies, comorbidities and general condition, is central to the adaptation of care. It is important to regularly assess disease progression, the effects of current treatments, and the patient's ability to tolerate therapeutic interventions.

- **Ongoing monitoring**: **Regular monitoring of** clinical parameters, such as vital signs, treatment tolerance and disease progression, can detect changes at an early stage. This monitoring is based on the use of appropriate assessment tools (biological analyses, imaging, clinical questionnaires) and constant dialogue with the patient.

- **Adjusting treatments**: Adjusting **drug** and drug-non **treatments** is a key component of adapting care. If a patient presents intolerable side effects or an inadequate response to a treatment, it is necessary to review the therapeutic strategy. This may include changing the dose, substituting the drug, or introducing complementary approaches such as physiotherapy or palliative care.

**Taking psychological and emotional factors into account**

Psychological aspects play a crucial role in disease management, particularly when the disease is chronic or progressive. Patients may experience feelings of anxiety, depression or emotional distress in the face of their evolving condition. These factors must be taken into account when drawing up a personalized care plan.

- **Psychological support**: **Psychological support** should be offered to patients who feel the need. This may include regular consultations with a psychologist, stress management techniques or support groups. Mental health is a key factor in treatment adherence and acceptance.

- **Empathic approach**: Caregivers need to adopt an attitude of **empathic listening**, providing a space where patients can express their fears, doubts and emotions. This approach helps to establish a relationship of trust and a better understanding of the patient's expectations, which is essential for adjusting care appropriately.

**Consideration of social and environmental constraints**

The patient's **social context** and available resources also influence management. Financial constraints, family obligations or lack of social support can limit a patient's ability to undergo treatment or access care.

- **Social assistance and logistics**: It is important to work with **social workers** or support services to help patients overcome these obstacles. This can include setting up home help, accessing funding for medication or medical equipment, or covering transport to care.

- **Family support**: Family involvement in care can be a valuable asset. Involving loved ones in the care process can help ensure better continuity of treatment at home, as well as daily emotional support for the patient.

## 2. Individualized treatment for optimal care

One of the pillars of adapted care is **individualized treatment**. Each patient responds uniquely to treatment, whether due to biological characteristics, environment or personal preferences. A tailor-made approach optimizes the effectiveness of care while minimizing adverse effects and meeting patient expectations.

**Customized treatments**

Advances in **personalized medicine** mean that treatments can be tailored to a patient's **biological characteristics**, such as genetic parameters, immune profile or risk factors. This is particularly relevant in fields such as oncology, where targeted treatments can better respond to tumor specificities.

- **Targeted therapies**: In cancers, for example, treatments can be tailored according to the tumor's **genetic markers**, providing greater efficacy and fewer side effects than conventional treatments.

- **Dose adjustment**: Some patients, depending on **age, weight, renal** or hepatic **function**, require dose adjustments to avoid toxicity while maximizing therapeutic effect.

**Non-drug approaches**

In addition to pharmacological treatments, **non-drug approaches** play a central role in adapting care. Functional re-education, behavioral therapies and relaxation techniques are invaluable tools for supporting patients in their care.

- **Rehabilitation and physiotherapy**: For patients suffering from musculoskeletal, respiratory or neurological pathologies, **functional rehabilitation** is essential to maintain or restore autonomy. Personalized exercise programs, under the supervision of physiotherapists, help reduce pain and improve mobility and quality of life.

- **Behavioral therapies: Cognitive-behavioral therapies** (CBT) can be used to help patients better manage the pain, anxiety or sleep disorders associated with their pathology. These approaches can help improve tolerance of treatment and adapt behavior in the face of the disease.

# 3. Flexibility and regular reassessment of the care plan

A care plan is never definitive; it must be **re-evaluated regularly** to remain relevant and adapted to the patient's needs. Changes in the patient's state of health, the appearance of new symptoms, or evolving personal preferences must be taken into account to adjust treatment.

**Continuous reassessment**

**Regular reassessment of** the treatment plan ensures early detection of any signs of disease worsening or the appearance of side effects. This relies on close clinical monitoring and close collaboration between the various healthcare professionals (doctors, nurses, physiotherapists, psychologists, etc.).

- **Clinical follow-up**: Regular medical check-ups, biological analyses and consultations enable us to monitor disease progression and treatment efficacy. This follow-up is essential for adjusting doses or modifying therapeutic approaches according to the patient's response.

- **Taking into account the patient's return**: The **patient's return** is a key element in the reassessment of the care plan. Patients are the first to feel the effects of their treatment, and should be encouraged to report any changes in their condition, whether improvement or deterioration.

**Flexible processing**

**Flexibility** is essential in adapting care. Treatments must be modified or discontinued if the patient does not respond as expected, or if side effects become intolerable.

- **Change of therapeutic strategy**: If a treatment is not producing the desired effects, it may be necessary to switch to another therapeutic strategy, whether by changing medication, combining several treatments or adopting a more conservative approach, such as palliative care.

- **Palliative care**: In situations where cure is no longer possible, **palliative care** offers an alternative focused on symptom relief and quality of life. Care in this context is adapted to meet the patient's physical and emotional needs, while respecting his or her end-of-life choices.

# 4. The importance of communication and coordination between healthcare professionals

Good **communication** between all members of the care team, and the patient him/herself, is key to **adapting care**. **Care coordination** is essential to ensure that all interventions are aligned and optimized for the patient's well-being.

## Communication between healthcare professionals

The care of patients suffering from complex illnesses often involves a multidisciplinary **team** of doctors, nurses, specialists, physiotherapists and psychologists. For care to be adapted and coherent, it is crucial that these professionals communicate regularly and share relevant information.

- **Consultation meetings**: **Multidisciplinary meetings** enable us to discuss the patient's progress and make joint decisions on treatment adjustments. This ensures that all perspectives are taken into account and that the patient receives the best possible care.

## Involving the patient in decision-making

**Patients** must be at the center of their own care plan. It's important to keep them informed at every stage, and to involve them in treatment decisions.

- **Informed consent**: Patients must be clearly and transparently informed about their options, including the benefits and risks of each treatment. A well-informed patient is more likely to actively engage in his or her care.

- **Taking preferences into account**: Patients' **preferences** in terms of treatment or quality of life must be respected. Some patients may prefer care that preserves their day-to-day comfort, even if this means limiting certain invasive treatments.

- **Technical aids and devices for patients with reduced mobility**
  - ○ Wheelchairs with integrated respiratory support, technical aids for oxygen therapy

**Wheelchairs with integrated respiratory support** and **technical aids for oxygen therapy** represent major advances in improving the quality of life of people with neuromuscular diseases, chronic respiratory illnesses or severe motor disabilities. These devices enable patients with specific respiratory needs to maintain their mobility and autonomy, while ensuring their respiratory safety. Integrating these aids into daily life is essential to guarantee optimum comfort, promote mobility and reduce the risks associated with respiratory insufficiency.

# 1. Wheelchairs with integrated respiratory support

**Wheelchairs with integrated respiratory support** are specially designed for patients with severe respiratory disorders, particularly those requiring continuous mechanical ventilation or oxygen therapy. These devices combine the need for mobility with adequate respiratory support, avoiding the need for the patient to be confined to a hospital or home environment to receive respiratory treatment.

**Key features**

Wheelchairs with respiratory support are equipped with features that facilitate both mobility and control of respiratory equipment. Here are some of the **main features of** these devices:

- **Support for assisted ventilation**: These wheelchairs can accommodate **non-invasive ventilation (NIV)** or **mechanical ventilation** devices, often required for conditions such as **amyotrophic lateral sclerosis (ALS)**, **muscular dystrophy** or severe **spinal cord injury**. The ventilator can be attached directly to the chair, allowing full mobility without interrupting respiratory treatment.

- **Portability of oxygen therapy systems**: these wheelchairs are designed to carry **portable oxygen concentrators** or oxygen cylinders, to ensure a constant supply of oxygen, even when on the move. They are equipped with special supports and secure storage compartments to avoid any inconvenience and guarantee patient safety while on the move.

- **Adaptive controls**: Wheelchairs for patients requiring respiratory support often include **customized controls**, such as joysticks or sip-and-puff systems for people with limited arm and hand mobility. These controls make it possible to maneuver the chair independently while receiving the necessary respiratory care.

## Benefits for patients

The **advantages** of wheelchairs with integrated respiratory support are manifold, particularly in terms of independence and quality of life. These devices enable patients to maintain a **level of mobility** while receiving essential respiratory care.

- **Greater autonomy**: One of the main advantages of these wheelchairs is that patients can move around without having to be constantly accompanied by a caregiver or healthcare professional to manage their respiratory assistance. This improves their **independence** and reduces the burden on family carers.

- **Respiratory safety on the move**: These wheelchairs enable patients to move around freely without interrupting their treatment. They are designed to prevent complications associated with respiratory failure, such as hypoxia, by guaranteeing continuous support during outings and daily activities.

- **Participation in social activities**: Thanks to combined **mobility** and respiratory support, patients can take part in more social, professional or family activities. This reduces the social isolation often associated with chronic or disabling diseases requiring ongoing respiratory care.

## 2. Technical aids for oxygen therapy

**Technical aids for oxygen therapy** are indispensable for patients with chronic respiratory diseases, such as COPD (chronic obstructive pulmonary disease), pulmonary fibrosis or neuromuscular disorders, who require prolonged or continuous oxygen supply. These devices facilitate the **day-to-day management** of oxygen therapy, ensuring a constant supply of oxygen at home or on the move.

### Types of technical aids

Technical aids for oxygen therapy can include several devices designed to make patients' lives easier and ensure effective respiratory management.

- **Portable oxygen concentrators**: These devices take in ambient air and concentrate the oxygen before delivering it to the patient. **Compact and lightweight**, they are designed for easy transport, enabling the patient to receive an oxygen supply even when on the move. Portable concentrators are often preferred to oxygen cylinders, as they do not require recharging and can operate continuously thanks to rechargeable batteries.

- **Mobile oxygen cylinders**: For patients who prefer to use oxygen cylinders, **lightweight, mobile versions** are available, designed for easy transport in a bag or cart.

These cylinders feature adjustable **flow regulators** to deliver oxygen at a controlled rate.

- **Mobility aids for oxygen therapy**: Devices such as **backpacks or carts** specially designed to carry oxygen cylinders or concentrators make it easier for patients to move around with their oxygen. These aids are essential for patients who wish to maintain a certain degree of mobility while undergoing treatment.

### Comfort and safety features

Technical aids for oxygen therapy integrate several functions designed to ensure both patient comfort and oxygen therapy safety.

- **Comfortable nasal cannula systems**: **Nasal cannulas** are often used to deliver oxygen directly into the patient's airways. Modern models are designed to be more **comfortable**, with soft materials that reduce nasal irritation and facial injury, even with prolonged use.

- **Alarms and monitoring systems**: Some oxygen therapy devices are equipped with **alarm systems that** signal a drop in oxygen flow, accidental disconnection or device failure. This ensures continuous monitoring and rapid intervention in the event of a problem, thus avoiding potentially dangerous situations for the patient.

- **Oxygen regulation devices**: Modern technical aids include **precise flow regulators** that adjust oxygen supply to the patient's specific needs, reducing the risk of under- or over-oxygenation. Automatic regulators can also adapt to the patient's needs, depending on his or her physical activity or state of rest.

**Benefits for the patient**

Technical aids for oxygen therapy provide a significant improvement in **quality of life** for patients with chronic respiratory needs.

- **Easier mobility**: portable concentrators and mobility aids enable patients to move around more freely while continuing to receive their oxygen, promoting independence and reducing isolation.

- **Increased safety**: Integrated alarm systems and monitoring features ensure safe care, reducing the risk of serious complications due to oxygen deficiency.

- **Comfort of use**: modern devices are designed to be **discreet** and **comfortable**, allowing prolonged use without discomfort. As a result, patients can continue their daily activities, including social and professional outings, with a minimum of discomfort.

  ○ Managing respiratory equipment in the context of disability

**Managing respiratory equipment in the context of disability** is an essential and often complex task, as it combines both specific medical needs and constraints linked to the mobility and autonomy of disabled people. People with motor, neuromuscular or other disabilities requiring respiratory assistance depend on sophisticated devices to ensure adequate oxygenation and effective ventilation. The use and maintenance of such equipment requires careful planning, training of patients and caregivers, and ongoing medical supervision.

# 1. Types of respiratory equipment adapted to disabilities

The respiratory equipment used by people with disabilities varies according to the underlying pathology and degree of respiratory dependency. These devices aim to compensate for respiratory deficits by providing support for ventilation or oxygenation.

**Non-invasive ventilation (NIV)**

**Non-invasive ventilation (NIV)** is a method used to assist breathing without the need for intubation or tracheostomy. It is often prescribed for people with neuromuscular diseases, such as **muscular dystrophy** or **amyotrophic lateral sclerosis (ALS)**, who suffer from progressive weakness of the respiratory muscles.

- **Positive pressure ventilation devices**: These machines deliver continuous or intermittent positive pressure into the airways through a face or nasal mask. They help the lungs to expand and maintain good oxygenation during sleep or exercise.

- **Customized masks**: Mask quality and comfort are paramount. **Custom-made** or adjustable **masks** minimize skin irritation and guarantee a good seal for effective ventilation.

**Mechanical ventilation**

**Mechanical ventilation** is used for people with **severe respiratory insufficiencies**, particularly in cases of diaphragmatic paralysis or after spinal cord trauma. This device can be used invasively (tracheotomy) to provide constant respiratory support.

- **Portable ventilators**: Modern portable ventilators enable people with severe disabilities to continue moving around and participating in daily activities while receiving

411

mechanical ventilation. These devices are compact, silent and battery-powered, guaranteeing safety even when on the move.

- **Alarms and monitoring systems**: The ventilators are equipped with **alarm systems** that signal any failure, oxygen desaturation or accidental disconnection, providing continuous monitoring and rapid intervention in the event of a problem.

**Oxygen therapy**

**Oxygen therapy** is often necessary for people with **chronic lung diseases** (such as COPD or pulmonary fibrosis) which limit the lungs' ability to deliver oxygen to the blood. In the context of disability, oxygen therapy systems need to be adapted to mobility requirements.

- **Portable oxygen concentrators**: Patients requiring continuous oxygen can use portable concentrators, which are more convenient than traditional oxygen cylinders. These devices draw in ambient air, filter and concentrate it to provide a continuous supply of oxygen.

- **Lightweight oxygen cylinders**: Mobile oxygen cylinders, often used with carts or backpacks, are practical for patients who don't move around a lot, or who need oxygen only intermittently.

**Secretion management devices**

For people with disabilities who have difficulty eliminating bronchial secretions due to muscle weakness, devices such as **cough-assist** or **bronchial suction** can be used.

- **Cough-assist**: This device helps expel secretions by generating positive pressure followed by negative pressure, which simulates the action of an effective cough, often absent in patients suffering from neuromuscular diseases.

- **Suction devices: Bronchial suction** systems are essential for clearing congested airways, especially for people unable to cough independently. These devices require specific training to avoid complications such as infection.

## 2. Daily management of respiratory equipment

The day-to-day use of respiratory equipment involves a number of tasks to ensure its proper functioning, as well as patient safety and comfort. **Training** of patients, families and caregivers is essential to ensure effective management and prevent complications.

### Training for patients and caregivers

**Initial** and ongoing **training** is needed to ensure that patients and their carers know how to use respiratory equipment correctly, manage alarms, and recognize signs of malfunction or worsening health.

- **Equipment use**: Caregivers must be trained in the **correct use** of ventilators, oxygen concentrators and suction equipment. This includes fitting and adjusting masks, monitoring oxygen flows, and managing alarms.

- **Equipment maintenance** : **Regular maintenance** is essential to keep respiratory equipment in good working order. This includes cleaning and disinfecting masks, tubes and cannulas, as well as replacing filters and consumables.

- **Battery management** : For portable devices, it's crucial to ensure that **batteries are charged before** going out or moving, and that spare batteries are available in case of failure.

413

**Planning and monitoring**

**Planning** and monitoring are essential to ensure that the use of respiratory devices is continuous and effective. This includes regular adjustments as the patient's condition evolves, as well as **medical check-ups** to reassess needs.

- **Follow-up visits: Regular visits with a pulmonologist** or respiratory specialist are necessary to monitor progress, adjust device settings and detect any potential complications.

- **Monitoring vital parameters**: Caregivers should monitor the patient's **vital signs**, including oxygen saturation, respiratory rate, and any signs of respiratory distress. Changes in these parameters may indicate the need to adjust device settings.

**Managing the unexpected**

Patients using respiratory devices need to be prepared for the **unexpected**, such as equipment failure or power cuts.

- **Emergency plans**: An **emergency plan** must be drawn up in the event of equipment failure, with clear instructions for contacting emergency services or using back-up devices. Mechanically ventilated patients should have access to a **manual rescue device** in the event of failure of the main machine.

- **Support network**: Caregivers and family need to know emergency numbers and who to contact for rapid troubleshooting of respiratory equipment, including technicians or oxygen suppliers.

# 3. Environmental adaptations for optimum use

Integrating respiratory equipment into daily life sometimes requires **adaptations to the home environment** to ensure that devices are easily accessible and functional.

## Home adaptations

The layout of the home to accommodate respiratory equipment must meet a number of requirements to ensure **comfort** and **safety**.

- **Accessibility of equipment**: Oxygen therapy and ventilation equipment must be placed in **areas that are easily accessible** to both patient and caregiver. Cables, hoses and other accessories must be securely stored to avoid the risk of falling or obstruction.

- **Electrical safety devices**: Respiratory equipment is often dependent on a power supply. It is essential to guarantee a **backup power supply**, such as an inverter or generator, in the event of a power failure.

- **Suitable storage space**: Equipment such as oxygen cylinders and concentrators must be stored in well-ventilated areas that comply with safety standards. **Organized storage** also ensures easy access to devices and consumables.

## Mobility adaptations

People with disabilities requiring respiratory support may need **specific adaptations** to guarantee their mobility and independence.

- **Wheelchairs with integrated respiratory devices**: These specialized wheelchairs enable patients to move around with their ventilation or oxygen device, offering **increased mobility** while ensuring respiratory safety.

- **Transporting devices**: If they have to travel frequently, patients may **need carts** to carry oxygen concentrators, as well as backpacks designed to hold portable oxygen cylinders. These mobility aids enable patients to remain active while undergoing respiratory treatment.

- **The caregiver as a player in respiratory care inclusion**
  ◦ Creating an inclusive, patient-friendly environment
**Creating an inclusive environment adapted to the needs of the patient** is a fundamental principle in the care of people with disabilities or chronic illnesses. This environment goes far beyond the physical or medical adaptation of the premises: it also encompasses psychological, social and relational aspects to ensure that the patient feels **valued**, **listened to**, and **autonomous** in his or her care. It is a comprehensive approach designed to reduce disability-related barriers, optimize access to care and improve quality of life. An inclusive environment recognizes the diversity of patient needs and implements strategies to meet them in a personalized and respectful manner.

# 1. Physical layout and accessibility

The first aspect of an inclusive environment concerns the **physical accessibility** of spaces, whether at home, in hospital or in public places. It is essential to eliminate architectural barriers and adapt infrastructures to facilitate movement and the use of equipment by people with disabilities or reduced mobility.

### Adapting home and care environments

**Adapting the home** is a priority to guarantee patients' independence on a daily basis. Medical equipment, mobility aids and practical adjustments must be designed to enable patients to move around and live comfortably at home.

- **Room accessibility**: It's important that living areas are **easily accessible**, especially areas such as the bedroom, bathroom and kitchen. **Wide doorways, clear** passageways and the absence of **steps** are essential elements to consider. The installation of **ramps or elevators** may be necessary in some cases.

- **Adapted bathrooms**: An **adapted bathroom** is crucial to guaranteeing independence in everyday gestures, such as toileting. This can include the installation of **grab bars**, **shower seats**, or **raised toilets**, to enable safe, independent use.

- **Functional room**: The **room** must be equipped with adapted furniture, such as a **medical bed** with electric height and tilt adjustments. Chests of drawers, bedside tables and other furniture must be easily accessible from the bed, especially if the patient has limited mobility.

**Accessibility in healthcare institutions**

In **healthcare institutions**, the environment must also be adapted to accommodate patients with special needs. This includes access to care, but also to all the services offered by the hospital or care center.

- **Clear, comprehensible signage**: A **signage system** must be in place to easily guide patients and their families around hospitals or care centers. This includes **Braille signs** for the visually impaired, and clear visual information to facilitate independent movement.

- **Access to medical equipment**: Examination rooms, consulting rooms and medical equipment must be designed to **facilitate access** for people in wheelchairs or with physical limitations. Medical devices, such as examination beds or imaging equipment, should be height-adjustable for easy use.

## 2. Empathetic, individualized approach to care

An inclusive environment is more than just architecture: it also incorporates a **human** and **empathetic approach** to care. Care must be patient-centered, respecting **individual needs**, rhythms and expectations. This relies on active listening and a relationship of trust between caregiver and patient.

### Active listening and patient empowerment

**Active listening** means paying attention to the patient's needs, fears and preferences, without judgment. It is essential that patients feel heard and respected, especially in the case of serious illnesses or severe disabilities.

- **Adapting to the patient's pace**: Support must be provided at a **pace suited to** the patient's abilities. This means not rushing care or decisions, but taking the time to explain each step and answer questions, in order to reassure the patient and establish an atmosphere of trust.

- **Respecting patient choice**: An inclusive environment values **respect for** patient **choice** and autonomy. If a patient prefers a particular approach to treatment or care, or has preferences in terms of comfort, these aspects must be taken into account and respected wherever possible. This includes **informed consent** for all interventions.

### Tailoring care to specific needs

Every patient has **different needs**, and an inclusive environment takes account of this diversity by tailoring care to the individual. It's not just a question of applying a standardized treatment, but of personalizing every aspect of care.

- **Multidisciplinary approach**: Treatment must be **multidisciplinary**, involving not only doctors and nurses, but also **physiotherapists, psychologists, social workers** and other specialists depending on the patient's specific needs. This ensures a comprehensive approach that takes into account physical, mental and social health.

- **Psychological and social support**: An inclusive environment also takes into account the patient's **psychological needs**. Anxiety, fear of the future, or difficulties in adapting to a disability can hinder acceptance of care. Offering **psychological support** is essential to help patients manage these emotional aspects.

## 3. Promoting autonomy and independence

Another fundamental pillar of an inclusive environment is the promotion of patient **autonomy**, whatever their condition. Even in situations of disability or chronic illness, it is possible to encourage independence through technical aids, rehabilitation and adapted solutions.

### Technical aids for mobility and daily living

**Technical** aids play a key role in empowering patients. They enable disabled people to regain a degree of independence in their day-to-day activities, reducing their dependence on caregivers.

- **Adapted wheelchairs**: **Electric** or manual **wheelchairs**, with features tailored to individual needs, enable greater mobility in the home and outdoors. Some models include respiratory support systems for people with chronic respiratory disorders.

- **Toileting and eating aids**: Devices such as **grab bars, seat raisers** or **adapted plates and utensils** help patients maintain **functional autonomy** when washing, eating or performing other daily tasks.

**Rehabilitation and reinforcement of autonomy**

**Rehabilitation** programs aim to maximize patients' residual abilities, whether to strengthen muscles, improve coordination or relearn certain movements after an illness or accident.

- **Functional rehabilitation**: **Physiotherapy** and **occupational therapy** are essential to help patients maintain or regain their independence. This may include muscle strengthening exercises, gait training, or learning techniques to compensate for loss of function.

- **Encouraging self-management**: An inclusive environment encourages **self-management** of illness or disability. This involves **therapeutic education** for patients, who must learn to manage their own treatment, diet and daily care, wherever possible.

# 4. Social integration and community support

An aspect often overlooked, but just as important, is the patient's **social integration**. An inclusive environment ensures that the person with a disability or chronic illness can maintain an active social life, and be included in the community.

**Participation in social activities**

It is essential to foster **social inclusion** by encouraging patients to participate in **group activities**, **leisure activities** or **community events**. Reduced mobility or physical limitations should not be barriers to social life.

- **Accessibility of public places**: To enable people with disabilities to participate fully in social life**, public places** must be accessible, whether by **ramps, elevators** or **adapted toilets**. Urban infrastructures must be designed to integrate all citizens, including those with special needs.

- **Adapted activities**: Offering **adapted activities**, such as sports classes for people with reduced mobility, or supervised outings, helps patients maintain an active lifestyle and stay connected to their social environment.

## Support for families and caregivers

Finally, an inclusive environment takes into account **caregiver** and family support. The caregiver's role is often an essential part of the patient's life, but it can also be physically and emotionally draining. It is therefore important to provide **support** and **resources** for family caregivers.

- **Psychological support for caregivers**: Offering **respite services** and **psychological support** to caregivers helps prevent burnout and ensures that they can continue to provide quality care while preserving their own well-being.

- **Family support**: Families need to be supported and trained to participate in the patient's inclusive environment. This includes **information sessions** on the patient's specific needs, the equipment to be used, and the care to be provided.

  - Supporting the autonomy of disabled patients

**Supporting the autonomy of disabled patients** is an essential objective in medical and psychosocial care. The aim is not simply to compensate for physical or cognitive limitations, but to promote the patient's independence, active participation and quality of life. This requires a person-centered approach, integrating personalized care, assistive technologies and an environment that encourages self-care. This autonomy support must be continuous and evolve with the patient's needs, taking into account his or her abilities, environment and life goals.

# 1. Understanding the concept of autonomy in disability

**Autonomy** is defined not only by an individual's ability to perform physical tasks without assistance, but also by his or her ability to **make decisions, actively participate in his or her own life**, and **manage his or her health** as independently as possible. For people with disabilities, supporting autonomy implies an approach that values participation, even if this is accompanied by support or technical aids.

### Recognizing abilities and limitations

To promote autonomy, it is essential to understand the patient's **residual abilities** and **functional limitations**. This helps to identify areas where the patient can act independently, and those where support or adaptation is required.

- **Assessing functional capabilities**: A precise evaluation of the patient's physical, mental and social capabilities is essential. This may include tests of mobility, muscular strength and balance, as well as cognitive assessments for people with neurocognitive disabilities.

- **Respecting self-determination**: One of our fundamental principles is to respect patients' **choices**. Even if the disability imposes certain limits, the patient must remain at the center of all decisions concerning him or her, including those relating to care, daily life and technical aids.

# 2. Promoting independence through technical aids

**Technical** aids play a crucial role in promoting the autonomy of disabled people. These devices, whether physical, digital or technological, enable patients to maintain functional autonomy in activities of daily living, whether at home, at work or in the community.

## Mobility aids

**Mobility** aids are essential for many people with disabilities. They enable independent movement, even for those with severe motor limitations.

- **Manual and electric wheelchairs**: **Wheelchairs** are one of the most important technical aids for people with motor limitations. Electric models, in particular, offer a high degree of autonomy, with customized controls adapted to individual needs (joystick, breath control, etc.). Some wheelchairs include built-in breathing devices for patients with respiratory disorders.

- **Walking aids**: Canes, walkers and other walking aids enable patients with **reduced mobility** to move around more safely and independently, both indoors and out.

- **Prosthetics and orthotics**: **Prosthetics** and **orthotics** compensate for motor deficits, improving the functional capacity of limbs or stabilizing weakened joints. These devices are often custom-fitted to optimize use and comfort.

## Assistive technologies for communication and daily living

**Assistive technologies** offer many possibilities for supporting autonomy in communication, care management and domestic activities.

- **Alternative communication tools**: For patients with speech impairments, **alternative communication** devices (such as apps or tablets with text-to-speech capabilities) make it easier to interact with others. These tools are crucial for people with cognitive or neuromuscular disabilities, as in the case of ALS (amyotrophic lateral sclerosis).

- **Home automation and connected objects**: **Home automation technologies** and **connected objects** are increasingly being used to make home management easier for people with disabilities. This includes voice control of lights, appliances, doors and even heating systems. These technologies enable patients to manage their environment without constantly relying on the help of a third party.

- **Healthcare applications**: **Care management** applications help patients to follow their treatments, monitor their vital signs, or schedule medical appointments independently. This encourages better health management and improves treatment adherence.

# 3. Rehabilitation and maintenance of functional capabilities

**Rehabilitation** is a fundamental pillar in supporting the autonomy of disabled people. By reinforcing remaining functional capacities or teaching compensatory techniques, rehabilitation enables patients to better manage their daily lives and maintain their independence for as long as possible.

### Physical and functional rehabilitation

**Functional rehabilitation** aims to maximize a patient's physical capabilities and compensate for deficits caused by illness or disability. It is based on collaboration between doctors, physiotherapists, occupational therapists and other healthcare professionals.

- **Physiotherapy**: **Physiotherapy** exercises help maintain muscle strength, balance and mobility, while reducing joint pain and stiffness. Physiotherapy is particularly important for patients with neuromuscular or orthopedic disorders, as it promotes independence in everyday movements.

- **Occupational therapy**: **Occupational therapy** focuses on improving independence in activities of daily living, such as dressing, grooming and meal preparation. Occupational therapists help adapt the patient's environment and develop strategies to compensate for functional limitations.

### Cognitive rehabilitation

For patients with **cognitive** or neurodegenerative **disorders**, cognitive rehabilitation plays a crucial role in maintaining mental and social autonomy.

- **Cognitive training**: **Cognitive training programs** help to improve or maintain functions such as memory, attention and planning. These programs are particularly suitable for people suffering from neurodegenerative diseases, such as Alzheimer's, or other cognitive disorders.

- **Memory aids**: **Technical aids** such as electronic diaries, medication reminder applications and alert systems enable patients with memory problems to manage their treatment and daily life more independently.

## 4. Create an environment conducive to autonomy

An **inclusive** and **adapted** environment is essential to promote the autonomy of patients with disabilities. This includes not only physical accommodations, but also social and psychological support, so that patients feel empowered to take charge of their own health and daily activities.

## Home improvements

To support autonomy, it's crucial that **home design** is adapted to the patient's needs, reducing obstacles to mobility and facilitating access to everyday management tools.

- **Accessible spaces**: Living spaces should be easily accessible, **with ramps**, **wide doorways** and **clear passageways** for wheelchair users or those with reduced mobility. The installation of grab bars in bathrooms or shower seats is also recommended to facilitate personal hygiene in complete safety.

- **Control devices**: **Home automation** systems and remote control devices enable patients to manage their environment (lighting, heating, electronic devices) without having to leave their homes, thus reducing their dependence on caregivers.

## Social and community support

**Social support** is just as important in encouraging independence. People with disabilities need to be included in social and community life, which can reduce isolation and improve psychological well-being.

- **Participation in social activities**: It's essential to encourage patients to take part in **group or** community **activities**, be they hobbies, adapted physical activities or social clubs. Not only does this help maintain an active lifestyle, it also boosts self-confidence and self-esteem.

- **Supporting caregivers**: Caregivers often play a key role in supporting the autonomy of disabled people. It is important to **train** and **support** them so that they can help patients effectively, while respecting their independence. Psychological support and respite services are also necessary to prevent caregiver burnout.

# 5. Encouraging self-care

**Self-care** is a central aspect of autonomy, especially for people living with a disability or chronic illness. Learning to manage one's treatments, medical appointments and day-to-day symptoms helps people to take better control of their condition and reduce their dependence on carers.

## Therapeutic education

**Therapeutic education** aims to empower patients to take charge of their own health, by teaching them to better understand their disease, recognize signs of worsening and know how to adjust their treatment accordingly.

- **Learning everyday gestures**: For patients requiring regular treatment (such as insulin injections, ostomy management or the use of respiratory devices), specific training courses can be organized to teach them how to perform these gestures independently.

- **Symptom monitoring**: Patients should be encouraged to **monitor their symptoms** proactively, using tools such as health diaries, mobile apps, or home monitoring devices (blood pressure monitors, glucose meters, etc.). This enables rapid intervention in the event of a problem, and avoids unnecessary hospitalization.

# Conclusion:

# Ethics and deontology in pulmonology

- **Ethical dilemmas in respiratory care**
  - ∘ Assisted ventilation at the end of life, limiting care

**Assisted ventilation at the end of life** and the **limitation of care** raise complex issues, both ethical and medical. These questions concern the management of respiratory symptoms in the last moments of a patient's life, the quality of the end-of-life experience, and respect for the wishes of the patient and his or her family. In this context, assisted ventilation may be an essential life support or a disproportionate intervention, depending on the medical circumstances and the patient's wishes. When the decision is made to **limit care**, the aim is to avoid aggressive or unnecessary treatment, and to focus on the patient's comfort and dignity.

# 1. Assisted ventilation at the end of life: purpose and role

**Assisted ventilation** involves providing mechanical support for breathing in patients unable to breathe sufficiently on their own. At the end of life, particularly in patients suffering from progressive or incurable chronic diseases (such as end-stage COPD, amyotrophic lateral sclerosis, or certain cancers), this respiratory assistance can pose dilemmas about its real usefulness.

**Purpose of assisted ventilation**

The main aim of **assisted** ventilation at the end of life is to maintain **adequate oxygenation** and reduce respiratory effort in patients with severe respiratory failure. However, in the terminal phase, when the patient's general condition deteriorates, the question arises as to whether this respiratory support is beneficial or unnecessarily prolongs suffering.

- **Prolonging life or improving comfort**: If assisted ventilation can prolong life, it is essential to ask whether it actually improves the **quality of that life**. At the end of life, the main objective should be to relieve suffering and improve comfort, rather than to artificially prolong an existence with no hope of recovery.

- **Reducing dyspnea**: Assisted ventilation, particularly **non-invasive ventilation (NIV)**, can sometimes be used to relieve **dyspnea** (difficulty in breathing), a frequent symptom in end-of-life patients. It can therefore play a role in symptomatic relief, even if the intention is not to prolong life.

### Types of assisted ventilation at the end of life

There are several types of **assisted ventilation**, which may be considered at the end of life depending on the patient's situation:

- **Non-invasive ventilation (NIV)**: Used with a nasal or face mask, NIV is a relatively less invasive method of supporting breathing. It can be used temporarily to reduce shortness of breath without requiring an invasive procedure, such as a tracheostomy. NIV can be a compromise at the end of life to maintain comfort without resorting to invasive measures.

- **Invasive mechanical ventilation**: In severe cases, **invasive mechanical ventilation** (via tracheostomy) is sometimes used to keep the patient breathing. However, at the end of life, this option is often considered excessive if the aim is solely to prolong life, with no possibility of improving the patient's condition.

## 2. Limiting care and ethics at the end of life

**Limiting** end-of-life **care** refers to the decision to restrict or stop certain medical interventions deemed unnecessary or disproportionate, such as assisted ventilation or other forms of intensive treatment. This approach is generally based on medical and ethical assessment, as well as on the wishes of the patient and family.

**Decision to limit care: criteria and discussion**

The decision to **limit care** is based on several criteria, including the medical prognosis, the potential benefits of treatment, and the patient's quality of life. These decisions are often taken after **in-depth discussions** between the healthcare team, the patient (when capable of expressing him/herself), and the family.

- **Prognosis and general condition**: When the patient's general condition is judged to be irreversible, and intensive care no longer offers any curative or significant benefit in terms of quality of life, limitation of care may be considered. This often concerns situations where the disease is advanced and incurable, and where survival depends solely on aggressive medical support, such as invasive ventilation.

- **Patient wishes**: It is crucial to respect the **patient's wishes**, expressed through advance directives or in discussions with caregivers. Some patients may choose to **refuse** invasive **treatments**, preferring a peaceful end of life free from unnecessary suffering. Respecting this wish is of fundamental ethical importance.

**Limiting or stopping assisted ventilation**

When the decision is made to limit care, this may include the decision to **stop assisted ventilation**, or not to introduce it if it is not already in place. This decision is particularly delicate and must be accompanied by strong **palliative support** to ensure that the patient does not suffer symptoms such as dyspnea when ventilation is stopped.

- **Palliative sedation**: In the event of discontinuation of assisted ventilation, **palliative sedation** can be used to alleviate the patient's suffering. This helps to reduce respiratory distress and pain, while accompanying the patient towards a peaceful end of life. Palliative sedation is administered when the aim is to relieve intractable suffering, not to prolong or shorten life.

- **Supporting the family**: Discontinuing care, including ventilation, can be a difficult time for the family. It is essential to offer **psychological support** and to explain the medical and ethical reasons for this decision, so that it can be accepted calmly.

## 3. Palliative care and comfort at the end of life

**Palliative care** takes on central importance in the context of a **care-limiting** approach. Its aim is to improve the patient's quality of life at the end of life, by controlling symptoms, reducing suffering and providing emotional and psychological support for the patient and family.

### Control of respiratory symptoms

**Palliative care** aims to relieve troublesome symptoms, particularly **respiratory symptoms**, which are common in patients at the end of life.

- **Oxygen therapy**: Low-flow **oxygen therapy** can be used to relieve breathlessness, even if the intention is not to prolong life. It can bring immediate comfort to patients suffering from dyspnea, without requiring full assisted ventilation.

- **Drugs to relieve dyspnea**: Opioids such as **morphine** are often prescribed in palliative care to **reduce the sensation of suffocation** and the anxiety associated with dyspnea. These drugs act by reducing the perception of respiratory effort and providing additional comfort.

**Holistic approach and support**

End-of-life care requires a **holistic** approach, taking into account not only physical symptoms, but also emotional, social and spiritual dimensions. Support must be centered on the patient's **dignity** and respect for his or her wishes.

- **Psychological support**: Patients at the end of life may experience anxiety related to imminent death or separation from loved ones. Psychological support is essential to help them manage this anxiety, and the presence of professionals trained in palliative care can ease this difficult transition.

- **Spiritual and family support**: Many patients at the end of life express **spiritual needs**, whether religious or not. End-of-life care can include spiritual support for those who wish it. In addition, it is essential to include the family in this process, providing emotional support and accompanying them through their own emotions and fears.

  ○ Balancing life extension and patient comfort

The **balance between prolonging life and patient comfort** is a central issue in medicine, particularly when it comes to patients suffering from serious chronic illnesses or at the end of life. This balance is based on complex decisions, which must take into account not only the patient's physical state of health, but also his or her **values**, **wishes** and **quality of life**. It is essential that healthcare professionals, in collaboration with the patient and his or her family, strike the right balance between **prolonging life** through medical treatment and maintaining the patient's **comfort** and **dignity**.

# 1. The dilemma between life extension and comfort

In medicine, there is sometimes a **dilemma** between offering care that could prolong a patient's life and that which aims to improve or maintain comfort. Intensive or invasive treatments, such as resuscitation, assisted ventilation or heavy chemotherapy, can in some cases prolong survival, but at the cost of reduced comfort, increased suffering, or degraded quality of life. This dilemma is particularly common at the end of life, when the disease is incurable and the benefits of treatment become uncertain.

**Life extension at all costs?**

**Prolonging life** at all costs, while possible with today's medical advances, is not always synonymous with a **better quality of life**. When treatments become cumbersome and invasive, and cause additional suffering with no prospect of significant improvement, the question arises as to their **proportionality**.

- **Aggressive treatments**: Some treatments, although effective in prolonging life, can be extremely demanding for the patient. For example, **prolonged invasive ventilation, repeated** chemotherapy sessions or complex surgical procedures can induce physical and psychological suffering, as well as making daily life difficult.

- **Benefits versus risks**: It is essential to assess the **benefit/risk ratio** of treatments. If the proposed treatment offers little chance of cure or significant improvement in general condition, but increases pain or discomfort, it may be ethical to reconsider whether to continue.

**Maintaining comfort at the expense of prolonging life?**

Conversely, some patients, particularly at the end of life or in the advanced stages of an incurable disease, may wish to prioritize their **comfort** and **quality of life** over prolonging painful survival. **Comfort** then **becomes** the priority of care, with medical decisions geared towards symptom relief and well-being, even if this means limiting certain potentially life-prolonging treatments.

- **Palliative care**: **Palliative care** is an essential part of this approach. It focuses on **symptom** management (pain, dyspnea, anxiety) and psychological and emotional support, without seeking to actively prolong life. The aim is to ensure a peaceful end to life, while **respecting the** patient's **dignity**.

- **Refusal of invasive care**: Some patients may decide to refuse treatments deemed too invasive, such as intubation, dialysis or chemotherapy, in order to concentrate on **daily comfort**. This decision is particularly common when the patient feels that his or her remaining quality of life is more important than prolonging survival.

## 2. The patient's values and wishes

At the heart of this consideration are the patient's **values** and **wishes**. Each individual has a different vision of what they consider a **good quality of life**, and these preferences need to be taken into account when making medical decisions. That's why it's vital to have open, honest discussions with patients as early as possible, to understand their priorities and expectations.

**Respecting the patient's wishes**

Respect for patient **autonomy** is a fundamental principle in medicine. This means that treatment decisions must be made in accordance with the patient's expressed **wishes**, whether through direct discussion, **advance directives**, or shared decisions with the family.

- **Advance directives** : **Advance directives** allow patients to express their wishes regarding medical treatment in situations where they would no longer be able to make decisions for themselves. This includes the choice of whether or not to continue assisted ventilation, resuscitation or other forms of life-prolonging treatment.

- **Ongoing dialogue: Ongoing dialogue** between the patient, caregivers and family is essential to clarify expectations and ensure that the care provided respects the patient's wishes. This allows treatments to be adapted as the patient's condition evolves.

## The importance of quality of life

For many patients, **quality of life** takes precedence over **quantity of life**. Quality of life is subjective and can vary from person to person. Some patients consider that a life marked by pain, complete dependence or loss of autonomy does not justify prolonging their survival through intensive treatment.

- **Subjective assessment of quality of life**: Healthcare professionals must take into account patients' perception **of** their own quality of life. For some, the ability to interact with loved ones, to communicate or to maintain a certain degree of physical comfort may be more important than survival itself.

- **Psychological support**: Patients need **psychological support** to enable them to express their needs, fears and anxieties in the face of end-of-life or heavy treatment. This support is essential to help them make informed and peaceful decisions.

## 3. The role of palliative care and support

**Palliative care** plays a key role in striking a balance between life extension and comfort. The aim of palliative care is not to cure, but to **relieve pain** and **symptoms**, while providing **holistic support** for the patient and family. Palliative care achieves this balance by addressing the patient's physical, emotional and spiritual needs.

### Symptom relief

One of the priorities of palliative care is to control **symptoms** that impact on the patient's quality of life, including **pain**, **dyspnea** (difficulty breathing), **anxiety**, and **digestive symptoms** (nausea, constipation).

- **Pain management**: **Pain management** is essential to ensure that patients can live out their final days in optimum comfort. **Opioids**, such as morphine, are often used to relieve severe pain, with doses adjusted to avoid excessive sedation or unnecessary side effects.

- **Palliative sedation**: In the event of refractory suffering (symptoms intolerable despite treatment), **palliative sedation** may be considered to relieve the patient by attenuating consciousness. This option is used as a last resort to ensure that the patient does not suffer in his or her final moments.

### Comprehensive, multidisciplinary support

Palliative care is a **multidisciplinary approach**, involving not only doctors, but also **nurses**, **psychologists**, **social workers** and sometimes **spiritual caregivers**. This holistic approach aims to support not only the physical aspects of illness, but also the emotional, social and spiritual dimensions.

- **Family support**: Family support is an essential aspect of palliative care. The patient's loved ones often experience moments of intense stress, anxiety and anticipated grief. Palliative care professionals help prepare the family for the patient's end-of-life, answer their questions and support them in their own emotional process.

- **Open communication**: **Communication** between the healthcare team, the patient and the family must be open, honest and empathetic. It is essential to clearly explain the options available, to avoid raising false hopes, while respecting the patient's wishes regarding the end of life.

- **Informed consent in pulmonology**
  ◦ Respecting the patient's wishes regarding treatment

**Respecting patients' wishes** regarding medical treatment is a fundamental principle of medical ethics. It is based on the recognition of patients' **autonomy**, i.e. their right to make informed decisions about their own health and treatment, in accordance with their values, beliefs and priorities. This respect for patients' wishes is particularly crucial in situations where invasive or life-prolonging treatments are envisaged, as well as at the end of life.

# 1. The principle of autonomy and informed consent

Respect for the patient's wishes is intrinsically linked to the principle of **autonomy**, which recognizes that every individual has the right to decide for themselves, according to their own values, about the care they do or do not wish to receive. **Informed consent** is one of the pillars of this principle, and means that patients must receive all the information they need to make an informed decision about their treatment.

**Informed consent: an ongoing process**

**Informed consent** is not simply an act of approval when a treatment is initiated. It is a **continuous process** in which the patient is informed in a clear, honest and comprehensible manner about :

- The nature of the proposed treatment.
- The expected **benefits** of treatment.
- **Risks** and potential **side effects**.
- Possible **alternatives**, including no treatment.

Once informed, the patient must be able to make a free, **unpressured** decision based on his or her personal values and priorities. This process enables patients to fully express their wishes and actively participate in decisions affecting their health.

**Patient decision-making capacity**

Respecting patients' wishes requires them to be able to make **informed decisions**. This presupposes that they have **decision-making capacity**, i.e. the ability to understand health-related information, to assess the consequences of their choices, and to communicate their decisions.

- **Impaired capacity**: In certain situations, such as dementia, severe cognitive impairment or acute confusion, the patient's decision-making capacity may be impaired. In such cases, decisions are made in collaboration with legal representatives or kin-of-next, always respecting the patient's **anticipated wishes** where known.

- **Advance directives**: Patients can prepare **advance directives** when they are still capable of making decisions, in order to express their wishes regarding treatment in situations where they would no longer be able to do so themselves. These directives, legally recognized in many countries, are an essential means of ensuring that the care provided respects the patient's values and preferences, even in the event of future incapacity.

## 2. Advance directives and end-of-life decisions

**Advance directives** enable patients to express their wishes in advance concerning the medical care they wish or do not wish to receive in circumstances where they would no longer be able to communicate their decisions. This written document reflects the patient's preferences regarding life-prolonging treatments, such as resuscitation, assisted ventilation or artificial nutrition.

### The content of advance directives

Advance directives usually include the patient's preferences on specific medical interventions, as well as general instructions on how he or she wishes to be treated in critical situations. Aspects often covered include :

- **Resuscitation**: Patients can express their wish to be resuscitated in the event of cardiac or respiratory arrest.

- **Assisted ventilation**: The patient can indicate whether he/she accepts or refuses **mechanical ventilation** in the event of acute or chronic respiratory failure.

- **Artificial nutrition and hydration**: Some people may wish to avoid **tube feeding or artificial hydration** at the end of life, especially if these interventions prolong survival without improving quality of life.

### Legal representative and medical power of attorney

In addition to advance directives, a patient can designate a **legal representative** or give **medical power of attorney** to a trusted third party. The role of this representative is to make medical decisions on behalf of the patient, should he or she lose decision-making capacity. It is therefore important that this person is fully aware of the patient's wishes and values, so that he or she can act accordingly.

- **Representative decision-making**: The representative must follow the **instructions** left by the patient in his or her advance directives, and if these are absent or imprecise, he or she must make decisions that respect the spirit of the wishes expressed by the patient during his or her lifetime.

## 3. Limitation of treatment and refusal of care

Patients have the right to **refuse treatment** that they consider disproportionate, unnecessary or contrary to their convictions. This right is fundamental and must not be called into question, even if refusing treatment could lead to a deterioration in the patient's state of health or death.

### Refusal of treatment

A patient can any refuse type of treatment, whether surgery, medication, chemotherapy or even **assisted ventilation** or **resuscitation**. Refusal of care can be motivated by a variety of reasons, including :

- The desire to prioritize **quality of life** over prolonging survival in conditions deemed unacceptable.
- Fear of treatment-related **side effects** or **suffering**.
- **Personal**, ethical or religious **convictions**.

### Limiting intensive care

In some cases, particularly at the end of life or in the face of an incurable disease, it is ethical and appropriate to limit intensive medical treatments that aim only to prolong survival without improving the patient's **quality of life**. This often includes decisions concerning :

- **Stop resuscitation**: If a patient has clearly expressed the wish not to be resuscitated, **DNAR** (Do Not Attempt Resuscitation) or **DNR** (Do Not Resuscitate) is applied.

This means that, in the event of cardiac or respiratory arrest, the medical team will not perform resuscitation.

- **Stopping or not initiating ventilation**: Similarly, a patient may decide to **refuse mechanical ventilation** in the event of respiratory failure, or the medical team may decide to limit this intervention if it is deemed disproportionate.

- **Stopping active treatments**: In some cases, it is possible to limit or stop active treatments such as dialysis, chemotherapy or artificial nutrition, if these treatments no longer bring significant benefit to the patient.

## 4. Ethical and communication considerations

Respecting a patient's wishes, especially at the end of life, sometimes poses **ethical questions** for caregivers. These decisions can be difficult, particularly when the family expresses different wishes, or when members of the medical team have differing opinions on what is appropriate to do.

### Open and respectful discussions

Decisions about limiting or withdrawing treatment must be **discussed openly and honestly** between the patient (if capable), family and caregivers. **Clear, empathetic communication** is essential to explain care options and their consequences.

- **Clarity and transparency**: Caregivers must provide clear explanations, free of complex medical jargon, of the implications of treatment decisions, so that patients and their families can understand what is at stake and make an informed decision.

- **Empathy and listening**: **Active listening** and empathy are important, respecting the emotions and opinions of all family members. Caregivers need to be sensitive to the emotional dilemmas that the patient's loved ones may experience, particularly in the event of disagreements between family members.

**Cultural and religious values taken into account**

Decisions about end-of-life medical care or intensive treatment are often influenced by **cultural**, **spiritual** or **religious values**. It is essential for caregivers to be attentive to these aspects, and to respect the beliefs of patients and their families wherever possible.

- **Spiritual care**: Some people may want spiritual support at the end of ,life such as the presence of a chaplain or religious leader, to help them make decisions in line with their deepest convictions.

  ◦ The caregiver's role in patient information

The **caregiver's role in patient information** is essential to medical care. Although the caregiver is not responsible for delivering complete medical information, he or she plays a crucial role as a **relay of information**, **mediator** and **source of support** for the patient. By being close to the patient on a day-to-day basis, the caregiver helps to create an **environment of trust**, where the patient feels listened to, respected, and well-informed about the practical aspects of his or her care. This not only improves **compliance with** treatment, but also alleviates worries and reinforces patients' **autonomy** in their care.

# 1. A close relationship with the patient

The **caregiver** is often the person who spends the most time with the patient during the day. This daily bond creates a **close relationship**, where the patient feels comfortable asking questions and expressing doubts or fears. This proximity gives the caregiver a **privileged position** to respond to certain requests for information and, in other cases, to identify information needs that need to be relayed to the nurse or doctor.

## Listening and observing

Thanks to their **constant presence**, caregivers are particularly well placed to **observe** patients and **listen to** their concerns. They can pick up on **verbal** and **non-verbal signals** that reveal misunderstanding, concern or distress, sometimes not expressed directly. By actively listening, he or she helps the patient to feel taken into account, and can then provide the practical information needed to clarify care.

- **Answering simple questions**: Sometimes, patients have simple questions related to daily care, such as hygiene gestures, the use of basic medical equipment (catheters, infusions, etc.), or taking medication. The caregiver can explain these practical aspects in clear, accessible terms, helping to demystify certain types of care.

- **Providing information on daily care**: Caregivers can also provide **simple explanations** of the actions they perform. For example, when toileting, he or she can explain why certain precautions are taken to prevent bedsores, or why certain hygiene procedures must be carried out in a particular way. This information, however basic, reassures the patient that **the care is justified**, and shows that he or she is not being kept in the dark about what is being done.

## Identifying information needs

By listening to the patient's needs, the caregiver also plays a crucial role in **identifying any gaps** or **misunderstandings** that may arise in communication between the patient and other members of the care team.

- **Relaying questions to the doctor or nurse**: If the caregiver realizes that the patient has questions that go beyond the scope of his or her skills, he or she can **relay** these concerns to the nurse or doctor. By acting as a **bridge between patient and caregiver**, questions can be answered appropriately, while respecting each person's area of expertise.

## 2. Clarification of medical instructions and treatments

One of the caregiver's roles is to ensure that the patient has fully **understood the instructions** given concerning his or her care, diet or treatment. This may involve **re-explaining** certain instructions given by the doctor or nurse **in a simple**, **accessible way**.

### Helping patients adhere to treatment

Sometimes, a patient may feel **lost** when faced with the complexity of the care or treatment they need to follow. The caregiver, by explaining **everyday gestures**, can help **facilitate the** patient's **adherence to** care.

- **Explain the purpose of medical procedures**: The caregiver can explain why it is important to perform certain procedures, such as regular mobilization to prevent bedsores, or the importance of following hydration instructions. This explanation helps to **motivate** the patient, who better understands the importance of following these instructions.

- **Help with medication management**: For patients who need to follow a strict medication regimen, the caregiver can explain how and when to take prescribed medication, and remind them of the instructions given by the nurse.

This is particularly important for the elderly or patients with cognitive impairment.

**Clarification of procedures and interventions**

In some cases, the caregiver can also explain **simple procedures** that are carried out on a daily basis, such as taking vital signs, infusions, or the use of certain medical devices.

- **De-dramatize care**: For patients anxious about care, such as taking blood or inserting a urinary catheter, the caregiver can play a **de-dramatizing** role by explaining the procedure, which helps to reduce the patient's anxiety.

# 3. Psychological and information support

As well as providing practical information, the nursing auxiliary also plays a **psychological** role. Their **emotional support** and caring presence are essential if patients are to feel at ease. The caregiver's human, empathetic approach enables the patient to feel at ease in expressing his or her **concerns** and **questions**, without fear of judgment.

**An emotional support role**

When faced with complex medical situations or information that is difficult to understand or accept (e.g., a serious diagnosis or heavy treatment), the caregiver provides local **psychological support**.

- **Active, sympathetic listening**: When patients receive important medical information, the nursing auxiliary is often the first to listen. By **listening sympathetically**, they enable patients to express their emotions, fears and misunderstandings.

- **Encouraging patients to ask questions**: Patients are often reluctant to ask doctors questions for fear of appearing ignorant, or for fear of the answers. By establishing a climate of trust, the caregiver can encourage patients to **ask questions** and **seek information**, reassuring them that it's legitimate to want to understand what's happening to them.

### Help interpret medical information

Even when the doctor or nurse has provided the patient with the necessary information, certain medical concepts may remain **abstract** or **difficult for** the patient **to understand**. The caregiver can then play a role in **interpreting** this information, using simpler language or repeating certain explanations in an accessible way.

- **Adapting medical language**: Medical vocabulary can sometimes seem complex. By knowing the patient well and observing his or her level of understanding, the caregiver can rephrase certain information in simpler words, adapted to the patient's level of comprehension.

- **Checking understanding**: The caregiver can also ask simple questions to ensure that the patient has understood the information given, and invite him or her to ask for further clarification if necessary.

## 4. Respect the limits of the caregiver's role

Although the nursing auxiliary plays an essential role in transmitting practical information and accompanying the patient, it is important that it **respects its limits** and **stays within its field of competence**. They do not replace the role of the nurse or doctor for complex information or medical decisions.

### Teamwork with nurses and doctors

The nursing auxiliary's role in patient information is always in **close collaboration** with the nurse and doctor. They must be able to **pass on** complex questions to the appropriate members of the nursing team, so as not to mislead the patient.

- **Working with the team**: Good **communication between members of the care team** is essential to ensure continuity and consistency in the information given to the patient. The caregiver must therefore ensure that any concerns or questions the patient may have are passed on to the team, so that appropriate responses can be provided.

- **Avoid giving unvalidated medical information**: Caregivers must avoid interpreting complex medical data or giving diagnostic or prognostic information that falls within the competence of doctors. He/she should always refer to competent professionals for questions that go beyond his/her remit.

- **Confidentiality and patient privacy**
  - Managing sensitive information

**Managing sensitive information** is a crucial part of the role of the caregiver and other healthcare professionals. It involves treating patients' personal and medical information with care and confidentiality, while respecting their right to **privacy** and **dignity**. Because of their regular contact with patients, carers are often on the front line when it comes to gathering sensitive information, which may concern health status, treatments or even personal and emotional aspects. This information must be handled with great care to protect the trust between the patient and the care team, and to comply with ethical and legal standards of **confidentiality**.

# 1. The legal and ethical framework of confidentiality

Sensitive information includes any data relating to a patient's state of health, diagnosis, treatments, but also personal and family data.

The management of this information is governed by strict privacy and data protection **laws**, such as the **General Data Protection Regulation (GDPR)** in Europe, as well as fundamental **ethical principles** in medicine.

**Professional secrecy**

As a healthcare professional, the nursing auxiliary is bound by **professional secrecy**, which means that it is strictly forbidden to divulge information concerning a patient to unauthorized third parties, except in specific situations provided for by law (such as an imminent danger to public health or judicial order). Professional secrecy covers all information shared by the patient in the course of care, whether of a medical or personal nature.

- **Privacy**: Caregivers must **protect** patient **privacy** by ensuring that medical and personal information is not shared with unauthorized persons, including other patients or relatives, unless the patient has given explicit consent.

- **Information shared with the healthcare team**: Within the medical team, information should be shared only with those professionals involved in the patient's care, and only to the extent necessary to ensure the quality of care.

**Medical data management**

Sensitive information relating to a patient's health must be handled with the utmost **discretion**. Access to such data must be restricted to authorized professionals only. This includes :

- **Digital data**: Electronic medical records must be protected by secure systems, and access must be strictly controlled by personal identifiers and passwords.

- **Written data**: Information contained in paper files must be **stored in secure**, locked cabinets, to prevent any leakage of information.

## 2. Building trust and managing personal information

The caregiver plays a key role in creating a **relationship of trust** with the patient, which is essential for quality care. This relationship often involves the patient sharing **sensitive information** about his or her health, fears, emotions or personal life. Managing this information with **respect** and **discretion** is essential to maintaining this relationship.

**Listening to and respecting emotions**

In the course of daily care, the caregiver may hear personal confidences, fears or sensitive questions from the patient. It is important for the caregiver to be **attentive** to this information and to respect the **emotional dimension** of these exchanges.

- **Caring listening**: The caregiver must **listen actively** and sympathetically, without judgment, to allow the patient to confide in them if they so wish. The aim is not to obtain information, but to be receptive if the patient chooses to broach certain sensitive subjects.

- **Managing emotions**: Sometimes, sensitive information concerns strong emotions linked to the illness, such as anxiety about death or psychological suffering. The caregiver can play a **calming role by** offering a place to talk, while remaining within his or her competence. If necessary, they can refer the patient to a competent healthcare professional, such as a psychologist.

**Transmission of relevant information to the team**

Some sensitive information may be of medical importance and must be passed on to other members of the health-care team. However, such information must be passed on **discreetly** and **appropriately**, respecting the principle of **necessity**: only information essential to the patient's well-being should be shared.

- **Relaying essential information**: If a patient expresses a major concern, or discloses a significant change in their state of health or living conditions that could affect their care, the caregiver has a duty to relay this information to the nurse or doctor to ensure complete care.

- **Protecting non-medical information**: All personal information that is not directly related to care, but which the patient has entrusted to us out of trust, must remain confidential and not be shared with the team, unless it has a direct impact on care.

## 3. Handling sensitive information with the family

The management of sensitive information concerns not only the patient, but also his or her **family** or close friends, who may sometimes be involved in medical decision-making or in supporting the patient. However, the caregiver must take care to respect the **patient's wishes** as to whether or not certain information should be shared with his or her family.

### Patient consent before sharing information

The patient has the right to decide which information can be shared with his or her family and which should remain confidential. Caregivers must always ensure that they have the patient's **explicit consent** before discussing his or her state of health or care with relatives.

- **Inform with caution**: If the family asks questions about the patient's state of health, the caregiver must be very **careful** not to reveal any information without the patient's authorization. They can give general answers about daily care (washing, eating), but for any medical questions, they must refer to the nurse or doctor.

- **Respect confidentiality**: If the patient has expressed the wish that certain information not be shared with his or her family (for example, a diagnosis of a serious illness), the caregiver must respect this wish and avoid any leakage of information.

## Managing tense situations

Sometimes, managing sensitive information can create **tensions** within the family, especially when relatives want to know more than the patient allows. In these delicate situations, the caregiver must remain **professional** and **diplomatic** in order to maintain the balance between confidentiality and communication with the family.

- **Emotional support for families**: Even without going into medical details, the caregiver can offer **emotional support** to the family, listening to their concerns and directing them to the appropriate professionals (doctor, psychologist) for more precise answers.

# 4. Digital privacy awareness

With the increasing use of **digital tools** in healthcare, the management of sensitive information also includes the protection of patient **computer data**. Caregivers, like all healthcare professionals, must follow strict protocols to ensure **data security** when using electronic systems to access medical records or record information.

## Digital best practices

It is essential that caregivers are trained in **best practices** for electronic medical record (EMR) management and data protection:

- **Secure access**: Always ensure that access to medical information is protected by secure logins and strict passwords.

- **No unauthorized sharing**: It is forbidden to share medical information by unsecured means (personal e-mail, unencrypted messaging). All sensitive information must be transmitted via secure channels set up by the healthcare establishment.

- **Deleting data after use**: When using computers or tablets for healthcare purposes, ensure that information is deleted or that you log out of the systems after use.

  ◦ Legislation and best practices

The **legislative framework** and **best practices** for managing sensitive information in the healthcare sector are essential to guarantee patient confidentiality and protect their personal and medical data. These principles are governed by specific laws in many countries, which impose strict obligations on healthcare professionals. In addition to laws, there are **best practices** that caregivers must follow to ensure that sensitive information is handled securely and respectfully.

# 1. The legislative framework for the protection of sensitive information

Patients' medical and personal information is considered **sensitive data** and must be protected in accordance with national and international laws. In Europe, for example, the **General Data Protection Regulation (GDPR)** imposes strict rules on how patient data must be handled. Other countries have similar legislation, such as **HIPAA** (Health Insurance Portability and Accountability Act) in the USA.

### RGPD (General Data Protection Regulation)

The **RGPD** is a legislative framework that protects the personal data of all people residing in the European Union. It grants rights to individuals with regard to the collection, processing and storage of their personal data, and imposes obligations on professionals who handle this data, particularly in the healthcare sector.

- **Explicit consent**: according to the RGPD, patients must give their **explicit consent** before their personal data is collected or used for medical purposes. This implies that healthcare professionals must clearly explain how the data will be used and why it is being collected.

- **Right of access and rectification**: Patients have the right to access their **medical records** and request rectification or deletion of inaccurate or unnecessary information.

- **Limitation of processing**: Personal data must be collected for **specific purposes** and may not be processed beyond these purposes without further consent. For example, medical information collected for an operation must not be used for marketing purposes without the patient's consent.

- **Data security**: The RGPD requires that **sensitive data,** such as medical records, be **protected** by appropriate security measures, such as encryption, restricted access, and secure IT systems.

**French data protection law**

In France, the **Loi Informatique et Libertés** has been in force since 1978, but has been adapted to comply with the RGPD. This law specifies the rights of individuals concerning their personal data and imposes specific obligations on healthcare professionals to guarantee the confidentiality of medical information.

- **Medical confidentiality**: In addition to the protection of personal data, **medical confidentiality** is a fundamental principle enshrined in law. It prohibits healthcare professionals from divulging information about a patient to unauthorized third parties, except in specific cases provided for by law (imminent danger, for example).

**HIPAA (Health Insurance Portability and Accountability Act)**

In the United States, **HIPAA** governs the way in which patient health information is protected. This law imposes security standards to protect **medical information** and guarantees patients' **right to confidentiality**.

- **Confidentiality**: HIPAA requires healthcare providers, hospitals and health insurers to take **strict measures** to protect identifiable health information.

- **Right to data portability**: Patients have the right to **transfer** their medical information between different healthcare providers, and healthcare organizations must guarantee this portability while ensuring data security.

# 2. Best practices for managing sensitive information

In addition to complying with the legislative framework, **best practices** play an essential role in protecting sensitive information. They concern both **digital** aspects (IT security) and **human** aspects (behavior of healthcare professionals). Here are just some of the best practices caregivers should follow to ensure the confidentiality of sensitive patient information.

**Respect for professional secrecy**

**Professional secrecy** is a key element in the relationship of trust between patient and caregiver. Caregivers, like all healthcare professionals, are bound by professional secrecy and must ensure that information concerning the patient's state of health is not shared with unauthorized persons.

- **Limit discussions**: Discussions about the patient's condition should take place in **private areas**, such as closed meeting rooms or offices, and not in corridors or public places where third parties could overhear confidential information.

- **Sharing information only with authorized persons**: Caregivers should only share sensitive information with members of the healthcare team directly involved in the patient's care. He/she must avoid divulging information to family members without the patient's consent, except in cases where this is necessary for his/her care.

## Protecting medical records

**Medical records** must be managed rigorously, ensuring that information is properly stored and accessible only to authorized personnel.

- **Secure storage**: Paper medical records should be stored in **locked cabinets**, accessible only by authorized professionals. Digital records should be stored in **secure computer systems**, with restricted access.

- **Controlled access**: All healthcare professionals must use their own **logins** and **passwords** to access IT systems containing sensitive information. It is important never to share these credentials with colleagues, or to use another person's credentials.

- **Systematic disconnection**: When a caregiver completes a consultation on a computer system or leaves a workstation, he/she must ensure that he/she is **disconnected** to prevent unauthorized access by a third party.

## Secure communication

**Sensitive information** must be **communicated** by secure means, whether between healthcare professionals or with patients.

- **Use secure channels**: To exchange sensitive medical information, it is important to use **encrypted e-mail** or secure platforms set up by healthcare establishments. We strongly advise against sending medical information via unsecured messaging systems or social networks.

- **Secure data transfer**: When it is necessary to **transfer** medical data between facilities or professionals, this must be done using secure transfer systems, such as secure messaging services or specialized healthcare data management platforms.

## Team awareness and training

Healthcare professionals must be regularly **made aware of** and **trained** in good practices for managing sensitive information. This training ensures that everyone involved in patient care fully understands their responsibilities with regard to **confidentiality**.

- **Regular training**: Healthcare facilities need to organize regular **training sessions** to remind people of privacy rules, new legal regulations and good data protection practices. This includes updates on cybersecurity risks, protection of medical records and incident management.

- **Culture of confidentiality**: It's important to promote a **culture of confidentiality** within teams, where every member is aware of the importance of protecting patient information and knows how to react in the event of a breach of confidentiality.

## Incident management

Despite the precautions we take, data breaches can still occur, either by mistake or as a result of a security vulnerability. That's why it's essential to have an **incident management plan** in place, so you can react quickly in the event of a problem.

- **Reporting breaches**: Any breach of confidentiality must be reported immediately to the competent authority within the healthcare facility. Under the RGPD, personal data breaches must be reported to the data protection authority within **72 hours** of discovery of the incident.

- **Corrective action**: After a data breach, it's important to implement **corrective measures** to prevent a recurrence. This may include revising security protocols, improving IT systems, or providing additional staff training.

www.ingramcontent.com/pod-product-compliance
Lightning Source LLC
Chambersburg PA
CBHW072132290526
45794CB00004B/1288